SOMATIC EXERCISES FOR HEALTHY HEART

A simple Step-by-step Guide to Stronger, Healthier Heart
and Overall Well-Being For All Ages

DR AVA M. RYAN

Copyright Page

Copyright © [2023] by Dr. Ava M. Ryan

TABLE OF CONTENTS

ADVANCE LEVEL

CONCLUSION

INTRODUCTION

An introduction to a healthy heart involves understanding the importance of cardiovascular health and the factors that contribute to maintaining it. The heart is a vital organ responsible for pumping blood throughout the body, delivering oxygen and nutrients to cells and removing waste products.

In the intricate landscape of human health, the heart stands as a beacon of vitality, tirelessly pumping life-sustaining blood through our bodies. This remarkable organ, nestled snugly within our chest, orchestrates a symphony of rhythms essential for our well-being. Understanding and nurturing the health of this vital organ is paramount for a fulfilling and vibrant life.

- **The Heart's Role in Well-being**

At the core of our cardiovascular system lies the heart, a muscular powerhouse responsible for circulating oxygen-rich blood to every cell, tissue, and organ in our body.

• Embracing Lifestyle Choices

The journey to a healthy heart begins with conscious lifestyle choices that prioritize cardiovascular health. Physical activity, balanced nutrition, stress management, and avoidance of harmful habits form the cornerstone of this journey.

• Exercise as Medicine

Regular physical activity is akin to a panacea for the heart, offering a myriad of benefits that extend far beyond the gym. From strengthening the heart muscle to improving circulation and lowering blood pressure, exercise is a potent elixir for cardiovascular health.

• Cultivating Emotional Wellness

In the garden of heart health, tending to our emotional well-being is as vital as tending to our physical health. Chronic stress, anxiety, and unresolved emotional burdens can cast shadows on our cardiovascular health, elevating blood pressure and increasing inflammation.

HOW SOMATIC EXERCISES PROMOTE HEALTHY HEART

Somatic exercises contribute to a healthy heart by indirectly supporting cardiovascular well-being. Through improved circulation, stress reduction, and enhanced flexibility, these exercises promote optimal heart health. By facilitating better blood flow and reducing stress levels, somatic exercises lessen the burden on the heart, lowering the risk of hypertension and heart disease. Additionally, fostering mindfulness and body awareness encourages individuals to make heart-healthy lifestyle choices, such as maintaining a balanced diet and managing stress effectively. Even during recovery from cardiac events, somatic exercises play a crucial role by rebuilding strength and restoring confidence in movement, ultimately supporting overall cardiovascular rehabilitation. While somatic exercises may not directly target the heart muscle, their holistic approach contributes significantly to maintaining a healthy heart and enhancing overall cardiovascular well-being.

BENEFITS OF SOMATIC EXERCISES FOR HEALTHY HEART

- **Improved Circulation**

Somatic exercises promote better blood flow throughout the body, including to the heart, which enhances cardiovascular health.

- **Reduced Stress Levels**

These exercises incorporate relaxation techniques, such as deep breathing and mindful movement, which help lower stress levels and reduce the risk of heart disease.

- **Lowered Blood Pressure**

By promoting relaxation and reducing tension in the body, somatic exercises can help lower blood pressure, a key factor in maintaining heart health.

- **Improved Posture**

By addressing muscular imbalances and promoting proper alignment, somatic exercises help improve posture, which in turn reduces strain on the heart and enhances overall cardiovascular function.

- **Support for Rehabilitation**

For individuals recovering from cardiac events or managing cardiovascular conditions, somatic exercises can aid in rehabilitation by rebuilding strength, improving mobility, and restoring confidence in movement.

- **Complementary to Traditional Exercise**

Somatic exercises complement traditional cardiovascular exercise by promoting relaxation, reducing muscle tension, and supporting overall well-being, making them valuable additions to a heart-healthy lifestyle.

ESSENTIAL TIPS FOR EFFECTIVE EXERCISE

- **Start Slowly:** Begin with gentle exercises and gradually increase intensity and duration over time to avoid exacerbating pain or causing injury.

- **Set Realistic Goals:** Establish achievable goals based on your current fitness level and health status. Gradually increase the intensity, duration, and frequency of your workouts over time as your fitness improves.

- **Listen to Your Body:** Pay attention to your body's signals and adjust exercises as needed to avoid overexertion or discomfort.

- **Warm Up and Cool Down:** Always begin your exercise sessions with a thorough warm-up to prepare your body for activity and reduce the risk of injury. Likewise, conclude your workouts with a cool down period to gradually lower your heart rate and promote recovery.

- **Stay Hydrated:** Drink plenty of water before, during, and after exercise to stay hydrated and support optimal performance. Dehydration can negatively impact your heart health and exercise performance.

- **Mix It Up:** Keep your exercise routine varied and interesting by trying different activities, such as hiking, yoga, or group fitness classes. Mixing up your workouts can prevent boredom and challenge your body in new ways.

- **Make It Enjoyable:** Choose activities that you enjoy and that fit your lifestyle, making it more likely that you'll stick with your exercise routine over the long term.

BASIC LEVEL

BRISK WALKING

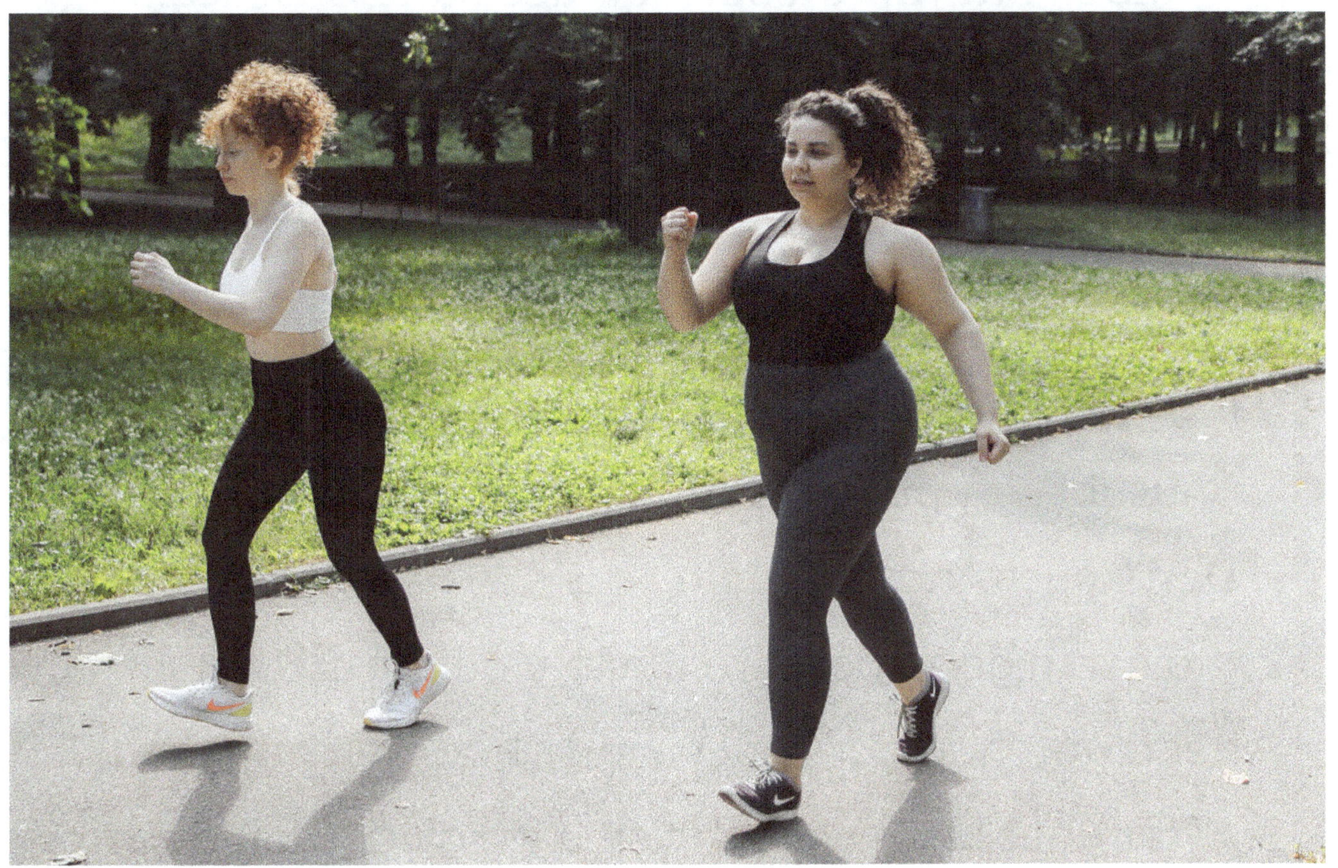

INSTRUCTIONS

- Stretch gently or walk slowly for a few minutes to prep your muscles.
- Comfortable, supportive footwear is key.
- Stand tall, shoulders back, and swing your arms naturally.
- Begin at an easy pace, then speed up to a brisk walk.

- Look out for uneven surfaces and obstacles.
- Bring water, especially in warm weather.

SAFETY TIPS

1. If you experience pain, dizziness, or any other unusual symptoms during your walk, stop and rest. Don't push through pain.
2. Maintain good posture while walking, with your head up, shoulders back, and abdomen engaged.
3. After your brisk walk, finish with a cooldown period to gradually lower your heart rate and stretch your muscles.

SWIMMING

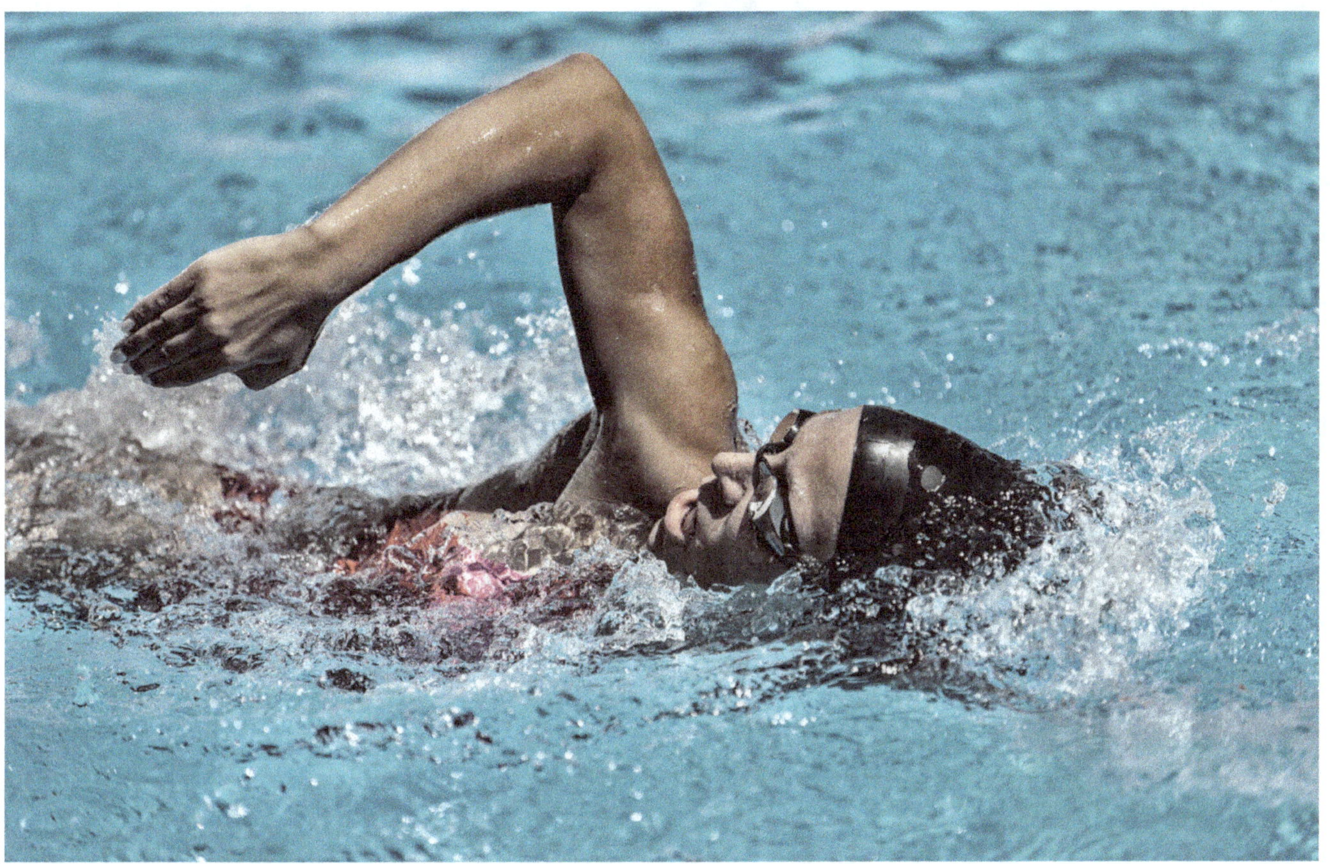

INSTRUCTIONS

- Start in shallow water, practice floating.
- Learn rhythmic breathing: inhale out of water, exhale in water.
- Learn Basic Strokes
- Focus on body position, timing, and coordination.

- Gradually increase duration and intensity of sessions.
- Practice regularly, set achievable goals.

SAFETY TIPS

1. Always swim in designated swimming areas supervised by lifeguards, if possible.
2. Swim with a buddy whenever possible.
3. Learn basic water safety skills, such as treading water and floating.

JUMP ROPE

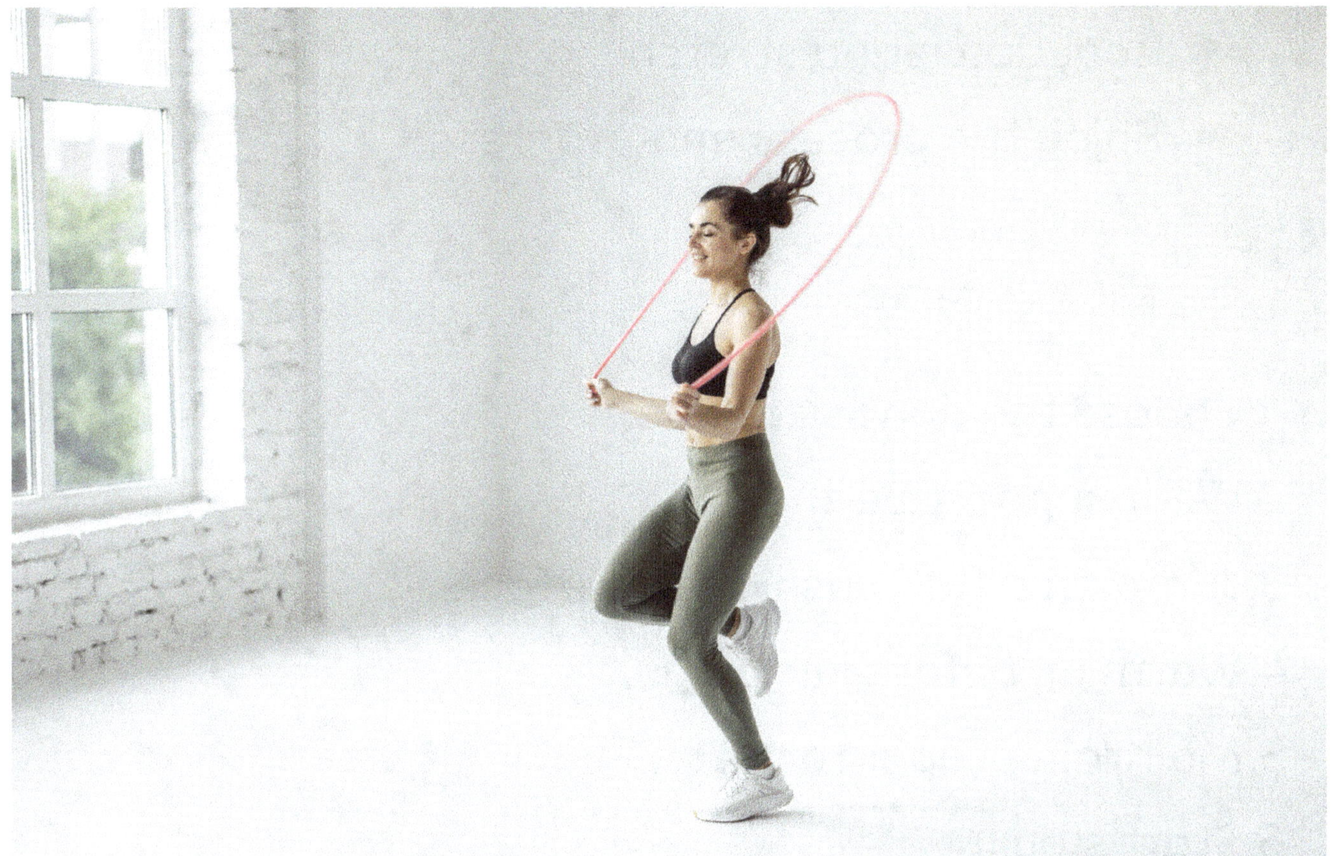

INSTRUCTIONS

- Choose the right length rope.
- Hold handles, swing rope with wrists.
- Jump as rope passes under feet.
- Start slow, focus on timing.
- Keep body relaxed, land softly.
- Practice regularly, increase duration.

- Try different techniques.
- Cool down and stretch.
- Enjoy the process and progress.

SAFETY TIPS

1. Choose the right size rope.
2. Wear supportive shoes.
3. Jump on a flat, cushioned surface.
4. Warm up before jumping.
5. Maintain proper form.
6. Start slowly
7. Stop if you feel pain.
8. Stay hydrated.
9. Take breaks.
10. Use proper technique.
11. Avoid overhead swings in crowded areas.

STAIR CLIMBING

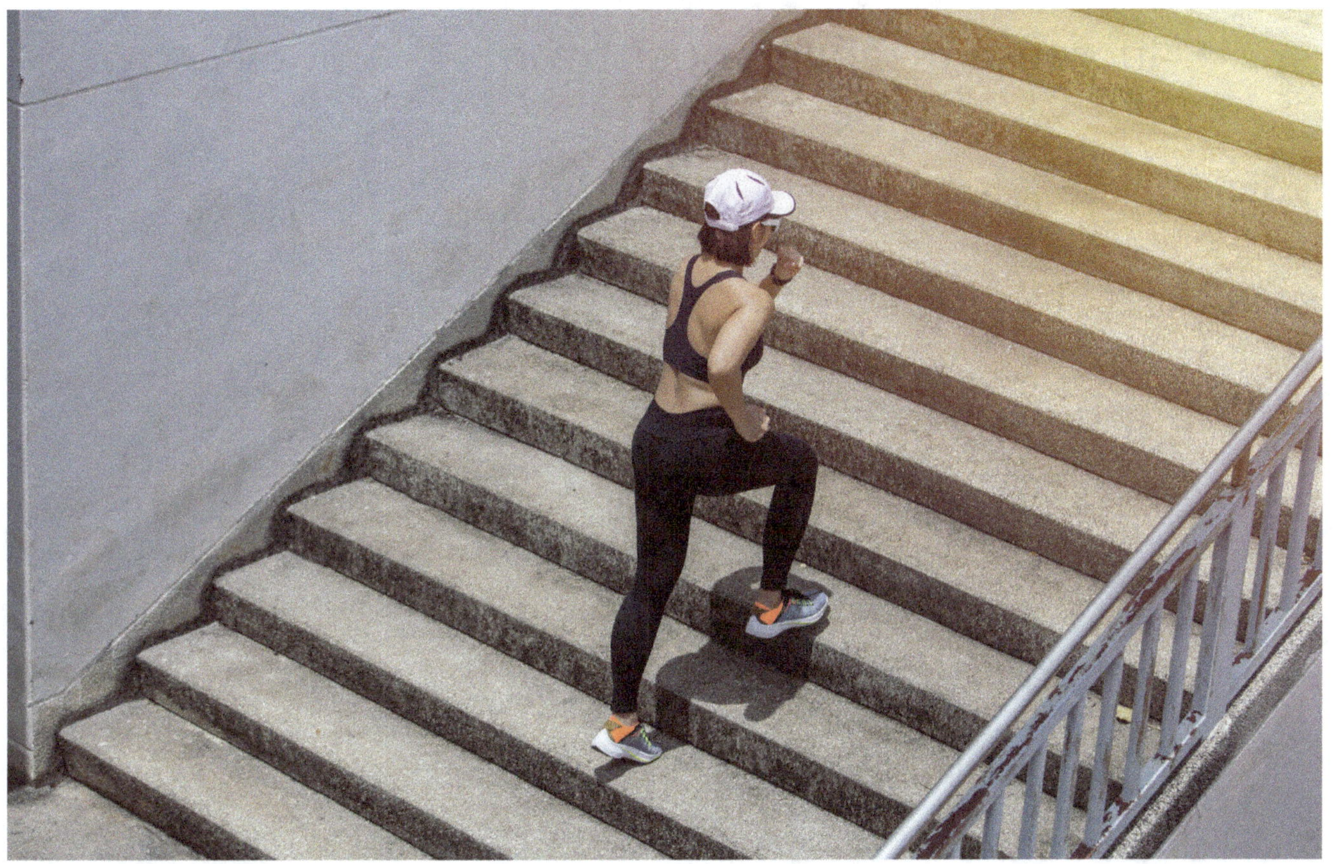

INSTRUCTIONS

- Find a set of stairs.

- Start at a comfortable pace.

- Use handrails if needed for balance.

- Step up one stair at a time.

- Keep a steady rhythm.

- Engage core muscles for stability.

- Take breaks if necessary.
- Increase intensity over time.

SAFETY TIPS

1. Wear good shoes.
2. Warm up.
3. Take one step at a time.
4. Keep good posture.
5. Stay focused.
6. Take breaks if needed.
7. Descend carefully.
8. Listen to your body.
9. Stay hydrated.

JOGGING IN PLACE

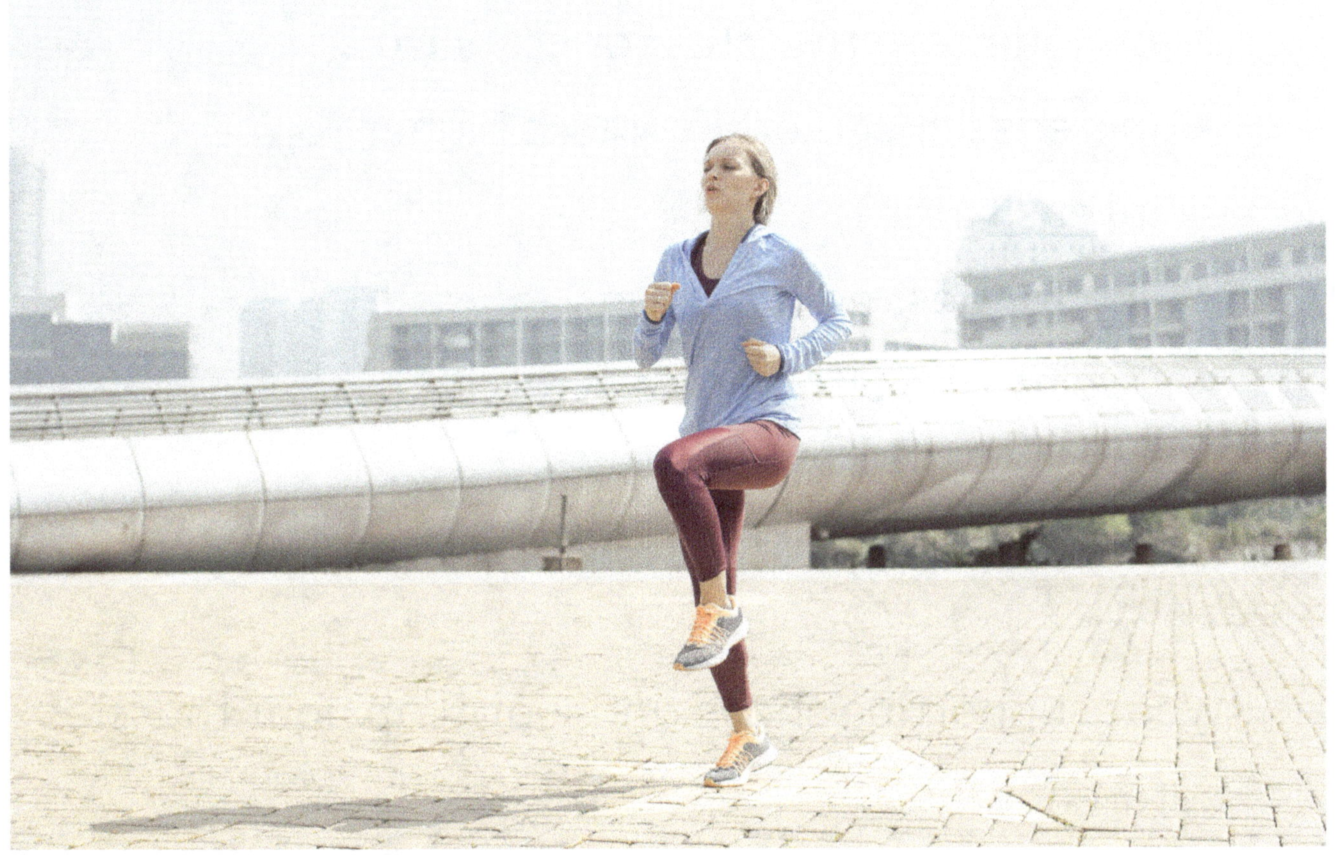

INSTRUCTIONS

- Stand with feet hip-width apart.

- Lift knees slightly, arms bent at sides.

- Begin jogging, lifting knees towards chest.

- Keep a light bounce, land softly on balls of feet.

- Swing arms naturally for balance.

- Maintain a steady pace.
- Engage core muscles for stability.
- Increase speed or lift knees higher for intensity.
- Jog for desired duration.
- Cool down with gentle stretches.

SAFETY TIPS

1. Wear supportive shoes and warm up your muscles beforehand.
2. Find a flat, stable surface to jog on.
3. Maintain good posture with your shoulders back.
4. Land softly on the balls of your feet.
5. Keep a steady rhythm.
6. Engage your core muscles.
7. Avoid over striding to prevent strain.
8. Listen to your body and pace yourself.
9. Stay hydrated throughout your workout.

STATIONARY CYCLING

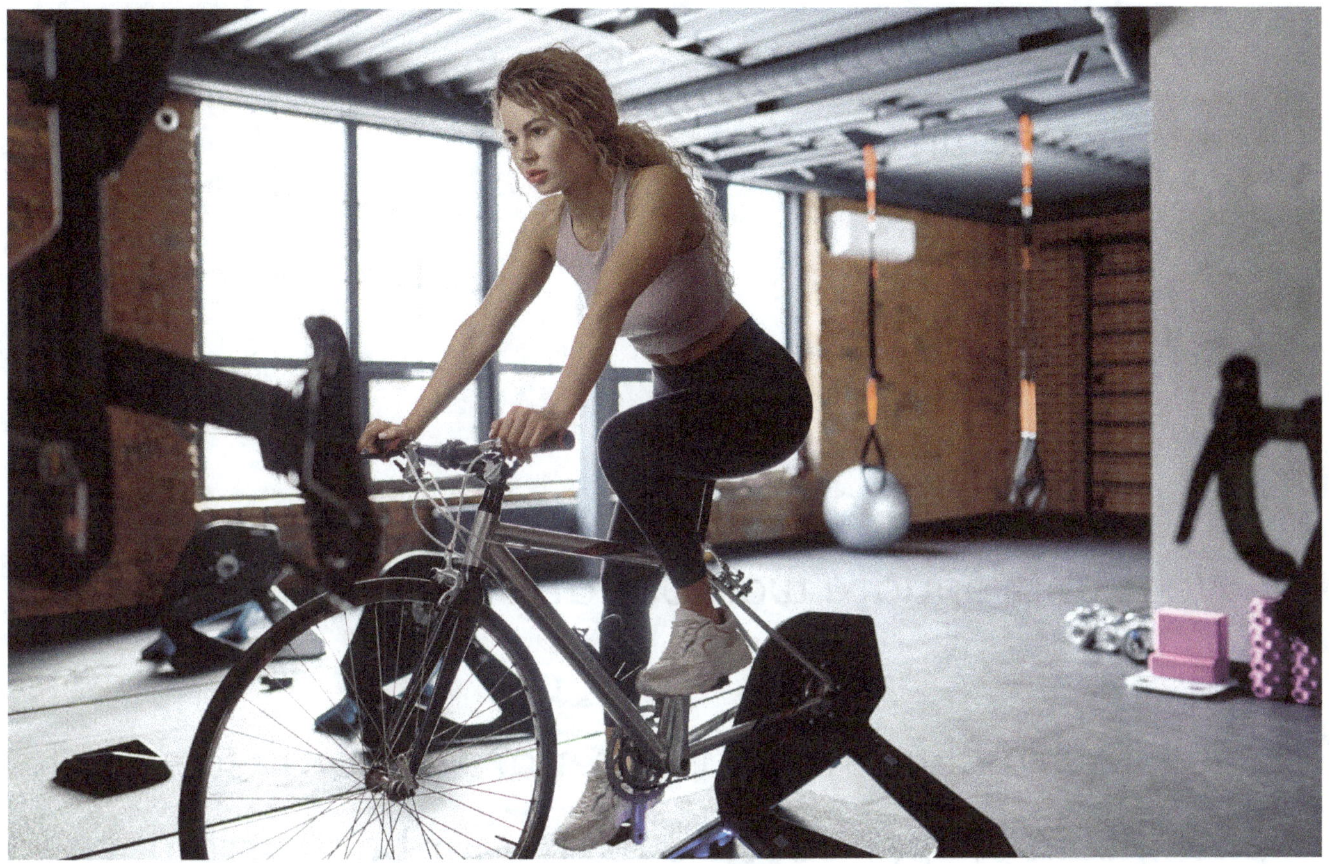

INSTRUCTIONS

- Set up the stationary bike.

- Adjust seat height and handlebar position.

- Start pedaling at a comfortable pace.

- Maintain good posture, keep back straight.

- Increase resistance for intensity.

- Pedal with smooth, controlled motions.

- Use handlebars for balance and support.
- Aim for a consistent cadence.
- Cool down and stretch after.

SAFETY TIPS

1. Adjust the bike to your size and comfort.
2. Wear appropriate workout attire and supportive shoes.
3. Start with a warm-up to prepare your muscles.
4. Maintain proper posture with your back straight.
5. Adjust resistance levels to match your fitness level.
6. Pedal smoothly, avoiding jerky movements.
7. Stay hydrated
8. Listen to your body.
9. Take breaks if you feel fatigued or dizzy.

DANCING

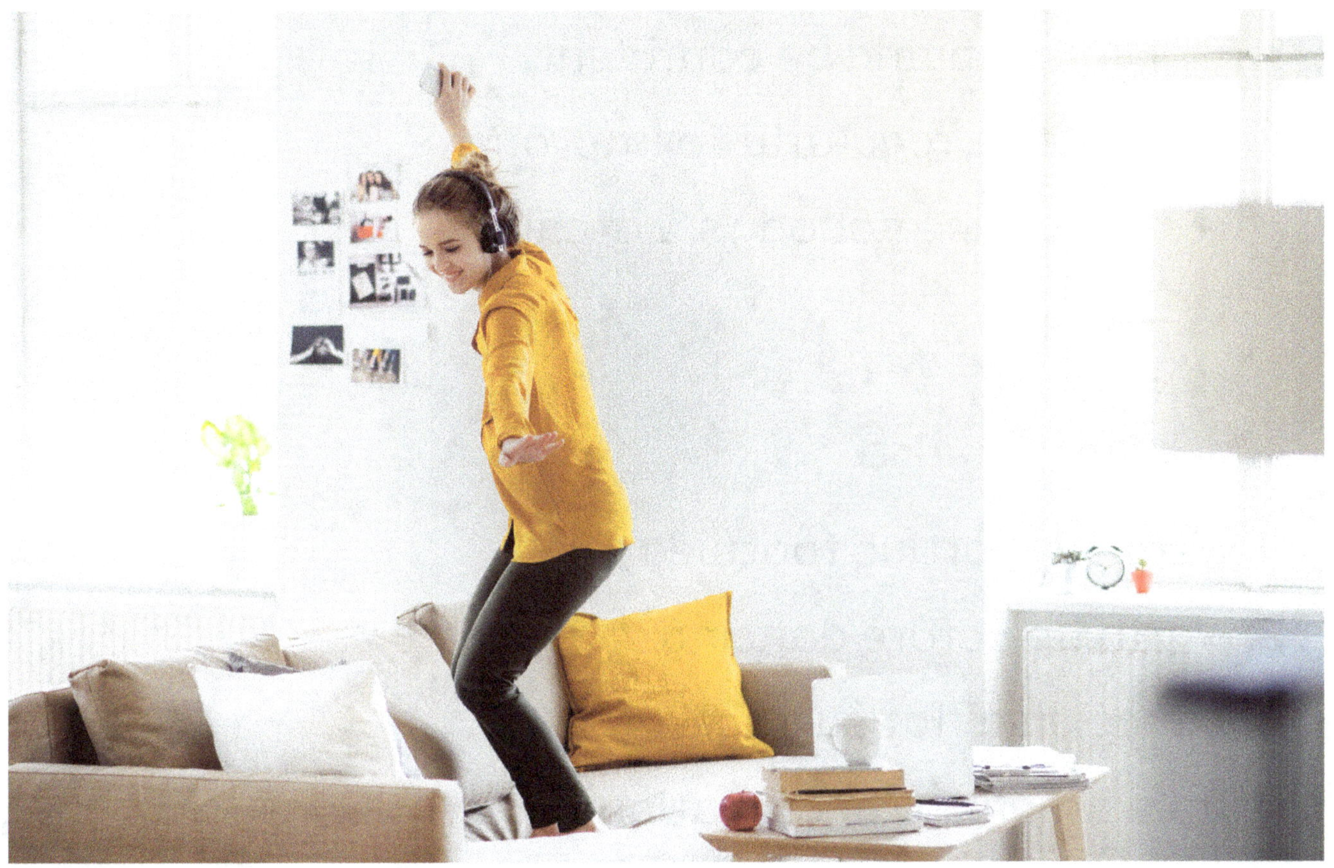

INSTRUCTIONS

- Choose your favorite music.

- Loosen up your body.

- Move to the beat.

- Let loose and express yourself.

- Pay attention to rhythm and timing.

- Use your arms, hips, and feet.

- Experiment with different styles.
- Have fun and be confident.
- Practice regularly to improve.
- Dance like nobody's watching!

SAFETY TIPS

1. Wear supportive footwear.
2. Warm up before dancing.
3. Dance on a flat surface.
4. Take breaks to avoid fatigue.
5. Stay hydrated.
6. Stop if you feel pain.

BUTT KICKS

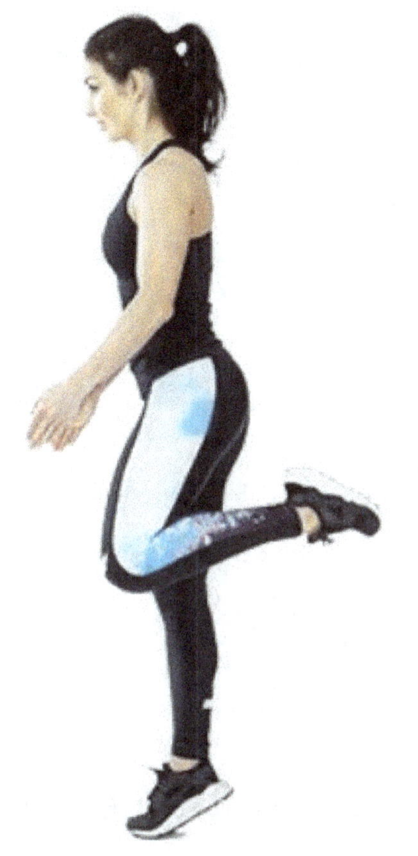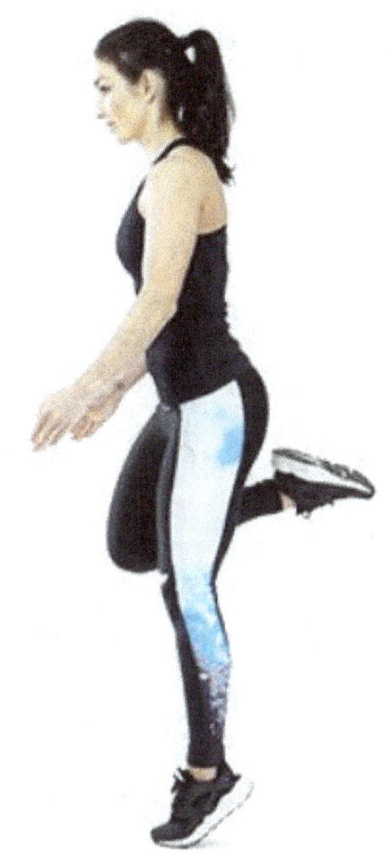

INSTRUCTIONS

- Stand with feet hip-width apart.

- Jog in place.

- Kick heels up to touch buttocks.

- Keep knees pointed downwards.

- Pump arms for momentum.

- Maintain a steady pace.

- Engage core muscles.
- Start with 30 seconds, increase duration.

SAFETY TIPS

1. Warm up before starting.
2. Start slowly
3. Keep your core engaged for stability.
4. Land softly on the balls of your feet.
5. Use your arms to help maintain balance and momentum.
6. Maintain a relaxed posture and avoid tensing up.
7. Stop if you feel any pain or discomfort.
8. Focus on proper form, kicking your heels up towards your glutes.
9. Keep breathing steadily throughout the exercise.
10. Cool down with stretches afterward to prevent muscle tightness.

JUMPING LUNGES

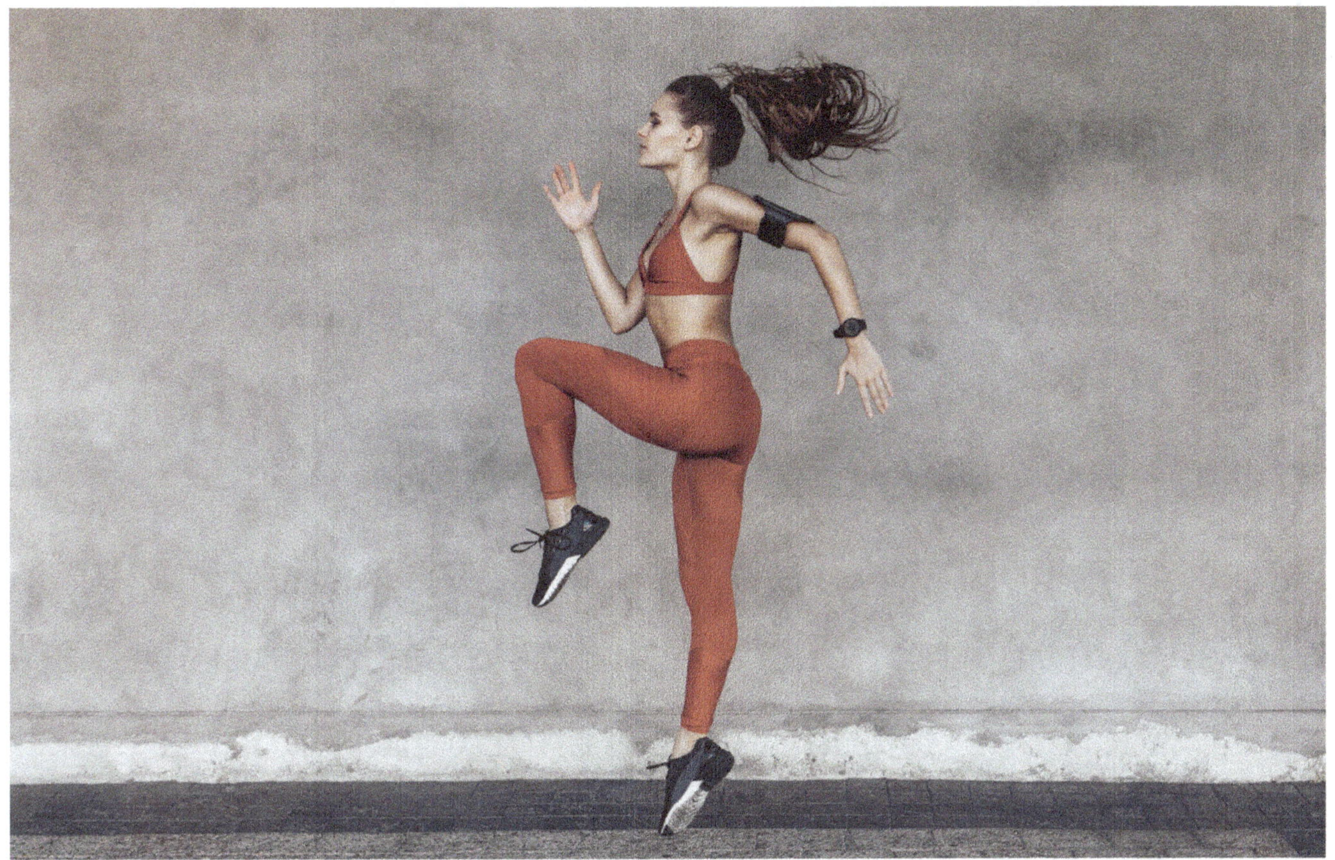

INSTRUCTIONS

- Start in a lunge position with one foot forward and one foot back.
- Lower your body until both knees are bent at 90-degree angles.
- Explosively jump up, switching the positions of your feet mid-air.

- Land softly in a lunge position with the opposite foot forward.
- Repeat the movement, alternating legs with each jump.
- Keep your chest up and core engaged throughout the exercise.
- Maintain a steady rhythm and controlled movements.
- Start with a few repetitions and gradually increase as you build strength and endurance.

SAFETY TIPS

1. Warm up.
2. Choose a flat surface.
3. Focus on good posture.
4. Start with small jumps.
5. Land softly.
6. Keep knees aligned.
7. Stop if you feel pain.

SHADOW BOXING

INSTRUCTIONS

- Find a clear space.
- Stand with feet shoulder-width apart.
- Keep hands up to protect face.
- Throw punches in the air.
- Alternate arms, stay light on feet.
- Incorporate footwork and head movement.
- Focus on form and speed.
- Visualize an opponent.
- Keep breathing and stay relaxed.

SAFETY TIPS

1. Warm up.
2. Use good shoes.
3. Engage core.
4. Start light.
5. Listen to your body.

PADDLE BOARDING

INSTRUCTIONS

- Get on the paddle board in calm water.
- Start on your knees to stabilize.
- Use the paddle to propel forward.
- Stand up slowly, keeping feet shoulder-width apart.
- Balance with knees slightly bent.
- Use core muscles for stability.
- Keep paddle close to the board for control.
- Relax and enjoy the ride.
- Practice turns and maneuvers.
- Stay aware of surroundings and water conditions.

SAFETY TIPS

1. Wear a life jacket.

2. Use a leash to stay connected to your board.

3. Check weather and water conditions beforehand.

4. Start in calm, shallow waters if you're a beginner.

5. Maintain proper stance and balance.

6. Keep a lookout for obstacles and other watercraft.

7. Use sunscreen and stay hydrated.

8. Learn basic paddling techniques.

9. Stay within your skill level and limits.

SEATED LEG PRESS WITH RESISTANCE BANDS

INSTRUCTIONS

- Sit on a sturdy chair.
- Loop resistance bands around feet.
- Place feet shoulder-width apart.
- Press feet against bands.
- Extend legs fully, but don't lock knees.
- Slowly return to starting position.
- Keep back straight throughout.
- Control movement for best results.
- Repeat for desired reps.

SAFETY TIPS

1. Warm up before starting.

2. Use a sturdy chair or bench.

3. Anchor resistance bands securely.

4. Sit tall with good posture.

5. Engage core muscles.

6. Start with light resistance.

7. Increase intensity gradually.

8. Listen to your body.

BOSU BALL JOGGING

INSTRUCTIONS

- Place Bosu ball flat side down.
- Step onto the center of the ball.
- Balance yourself with arms out.
- Begin jogging in place.
- Keep movements controlled.
- Engage core for stability.
- Start with slow pace.
- Gradually increase speed.
- Focus on balance and coordination.

SAFETY TIPS

1. Warm up before using the Bosu ball.
2. Place the Bosu ball on a stable surface.
3. Wear supportive shoes.
4. Maintain a steady rhythm.
5. Listen to your body.

INTERMEDIATE LEVEL

BURPEES

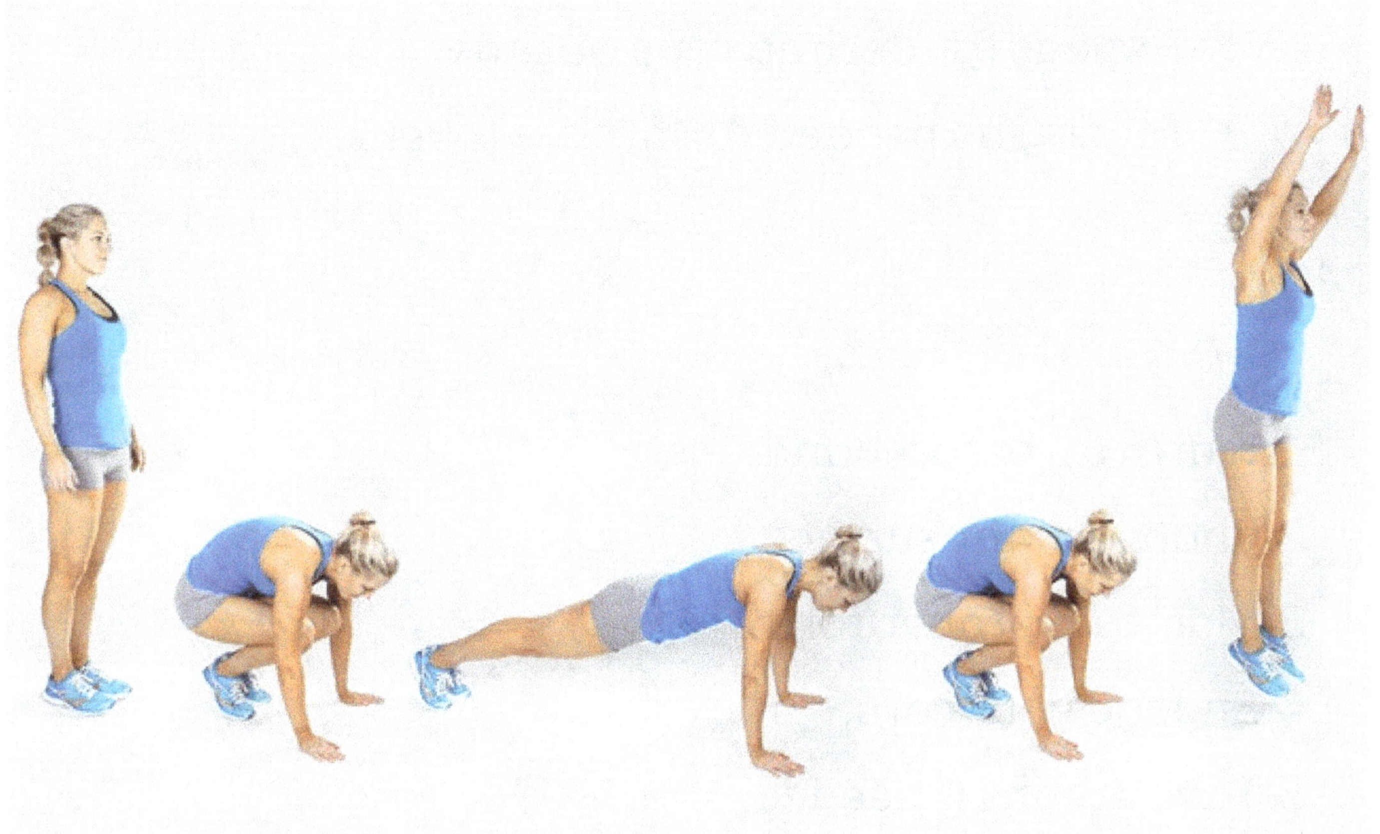

INSTRUCTIONS

- Start in a standing position.

- Drop into a squat, hands on the floor.

- Kick feet back into a plank.

- Lower chest to the floor.

- Push back up to plank position.

- Jump feet back to hands.

- Explode into a jump with arms raised.
- Repeat for desired reps or time.
- Modify as needed for fitness level.

SAFETY TIPS

1. Warm up beforehand.
2. Choose a flat surface.
3. Maintain proper form.
4. Engage your core.
5. Take breaks if needed.
6. Listen to your body.
7. Stay hydrated.

SIDE PLANK

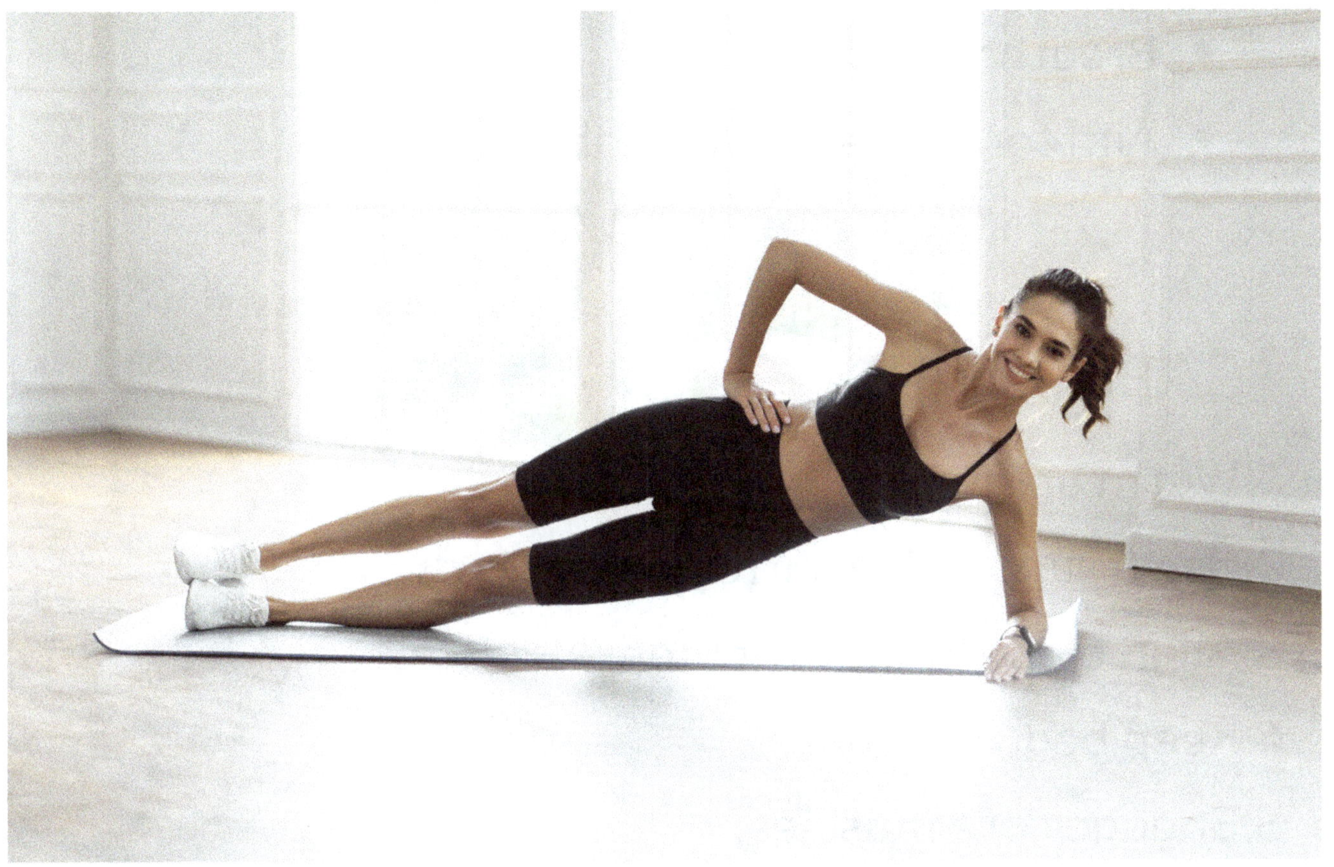

INSTRUCTIONS

- Lie on your side.

- Support your body with one forearm.

- Lift your hips off the ground.

- Keep your body straight.

- Hold for desired time.

- Switch sides.

- Engage core muscles.
- Breathe steadily.
- Aim for balance and stability.

SAFETY TIPS

1. Warm up first.
2. Use a supportive surface.
3. Align elbow under shoulder.
4. Keep body straight.
5. Engage core muscles.
6. Lift hips into position.
7. Focus on balance.
8. Breathe steadily.

MOUNTAIN CLIMBERS

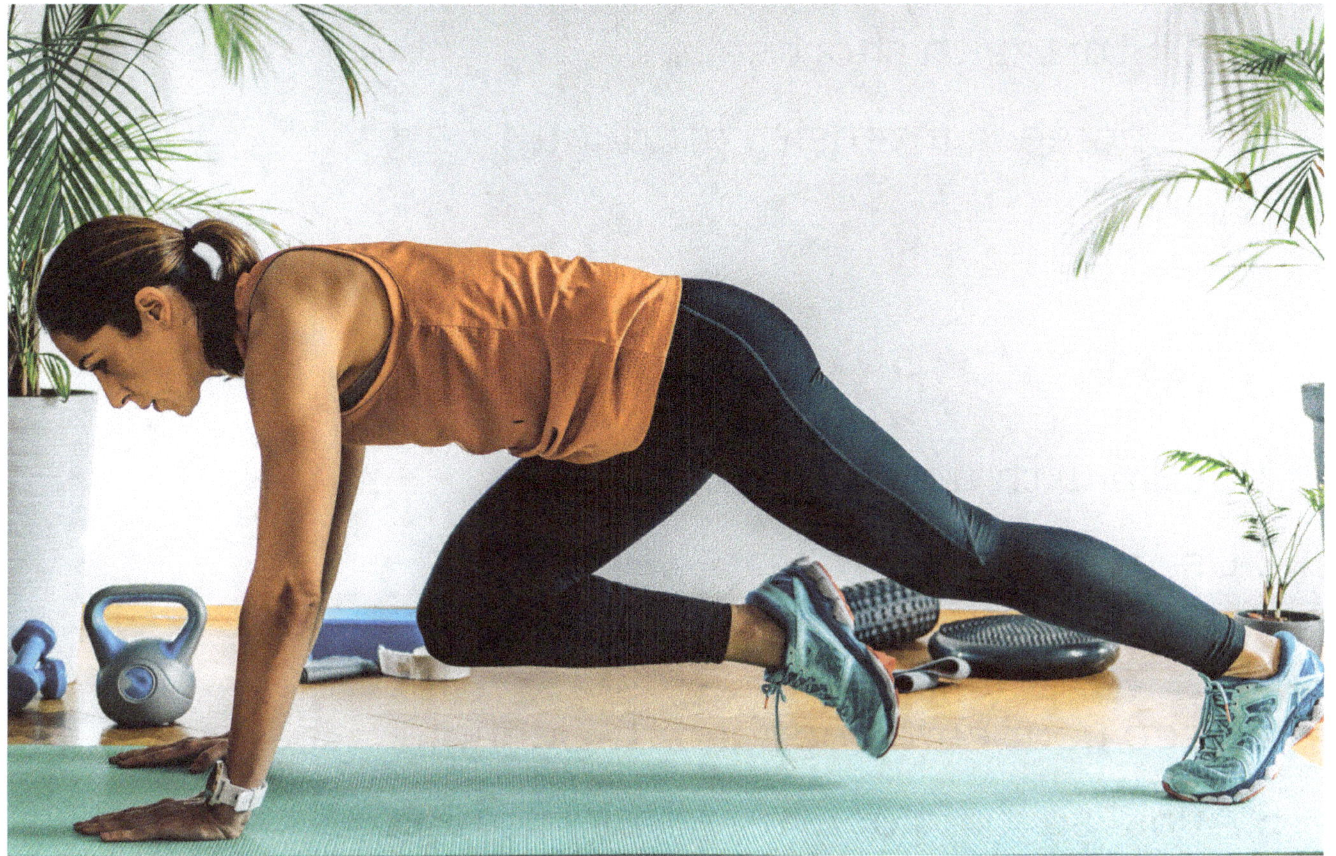

INSTRUCTIONS

- Start in a plank position.

- Bring one knee towards your chest.

- Alternate legs quickly.

- Keep your core engaged.

- Maintain a steady pace.

- Aim for full range of motion.

- Breathe steadily throughout.
- Start with short sets.
- Increase intensity gradually.

SAFETY TIPS

1. Begin with a proper warm-up.
2. Use a stable surface.
3. Start in a high plank position.
4. Keep your core engaged throughout.
5. Avoid sagging or lifting hips too high.
6. Focus on breathing rhythmically.
7. Listen to your body
8. Modify the exercise if it causes discomfort.

HIGH KNEES

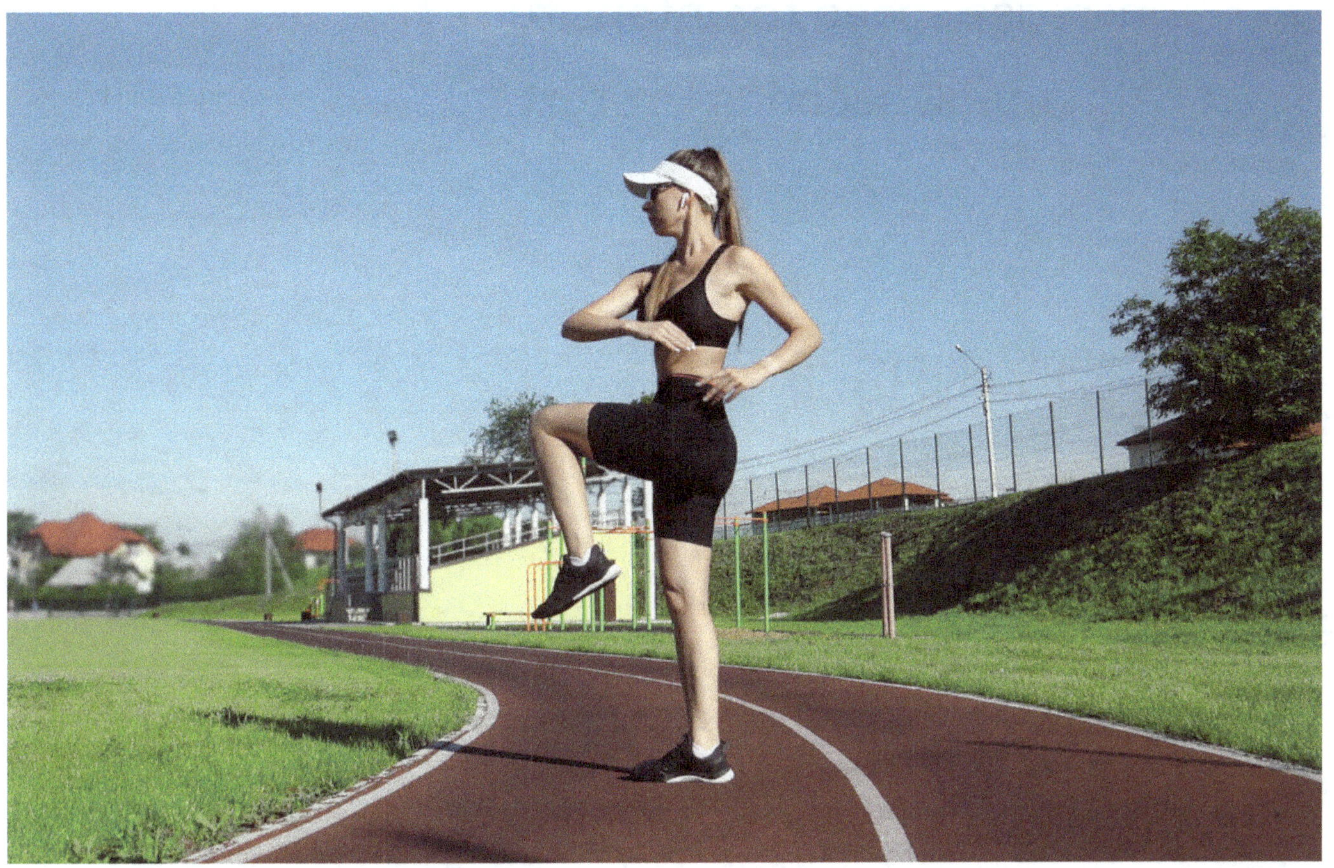

INSTRUCTIONS

- Stand tall with feet hip-width apart.
- Lift one knee towards chest.
- Alternate quickly, pumping arms.
- Aim for knee height or higher.
- Stay light on feet, land softly.
- Keep core engaged for balance.

- Increase speed for intensity.
- Aim for 30 seconds to start.

SAFETY TIPS

1. Warm up
2. Engage core muscles.
3. Lift knees high.
4. Keep back straight.
5. Land softly.
6. Use arms for momentum.
7. Start slowly.
8. Take breaks if needed.
9. Stay hydrated.

RUSSIAN TWIST

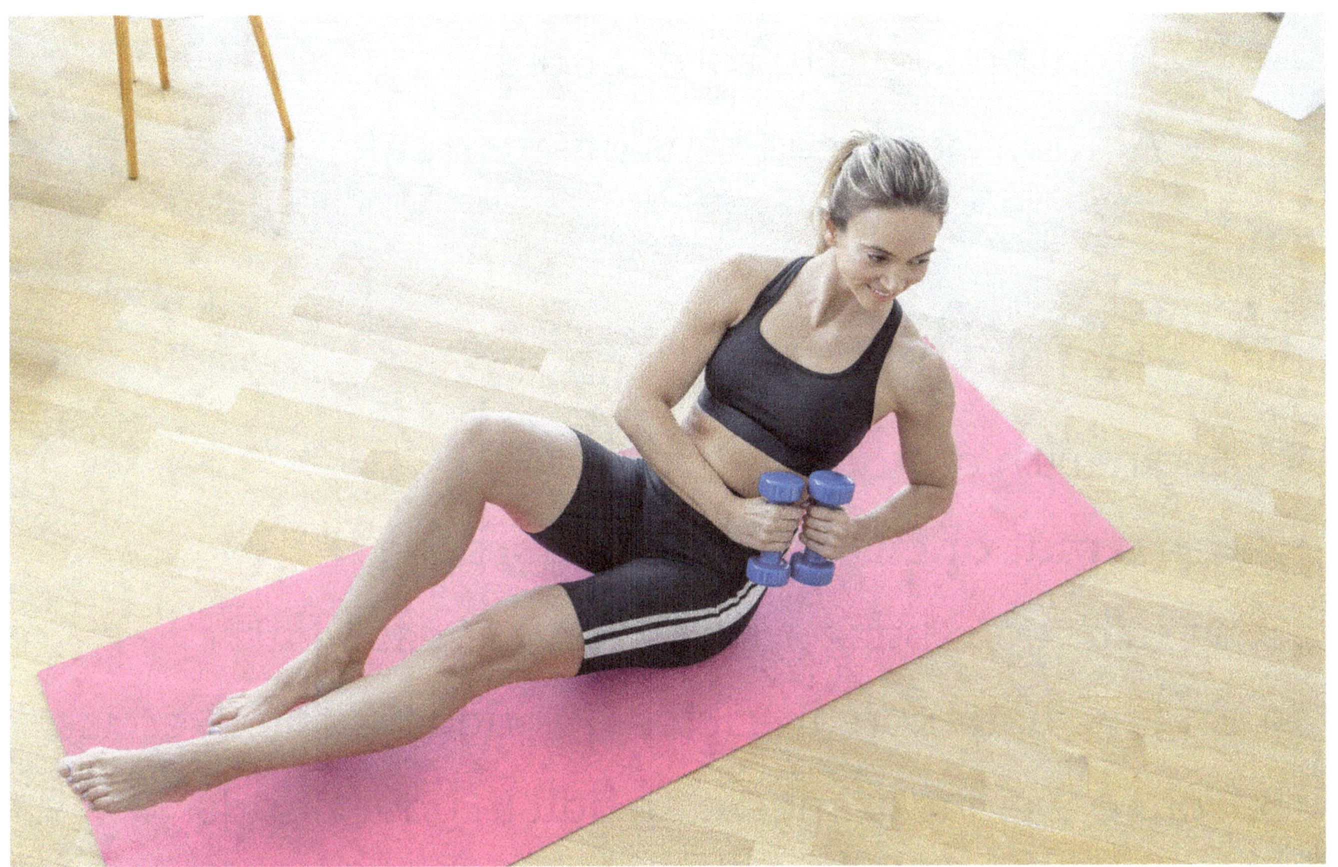

INSTRUCTIONS

- Sit on the floor, knees bent.

- Lean back slightly, engage core.

- Hold a weight or medicine ball.

- Twist torso to one side, touch floor.

- Return to center, then twist other side.

- Keep movements controlled.

- Focus on core engagement.
- Breathe steadily throughout.
- Aim for balanced reps on each side.

SAFETY TIPS

1. Begin with a proper warm-up.
2. Use a mat or cushion for support.
3. Sit with your back straight and knees bent.
4. Engage your core muscles throughout the exercise.
5. Hold a weight or medicine ball in your hands.
6. Avoid rounding your back or straining your neck.
7. Exhale as you twist to fully engage your abdominals.
8. Start with lighter weights.
9. Listen to your body and stop if you feel any discomfort.

PUSHUPS

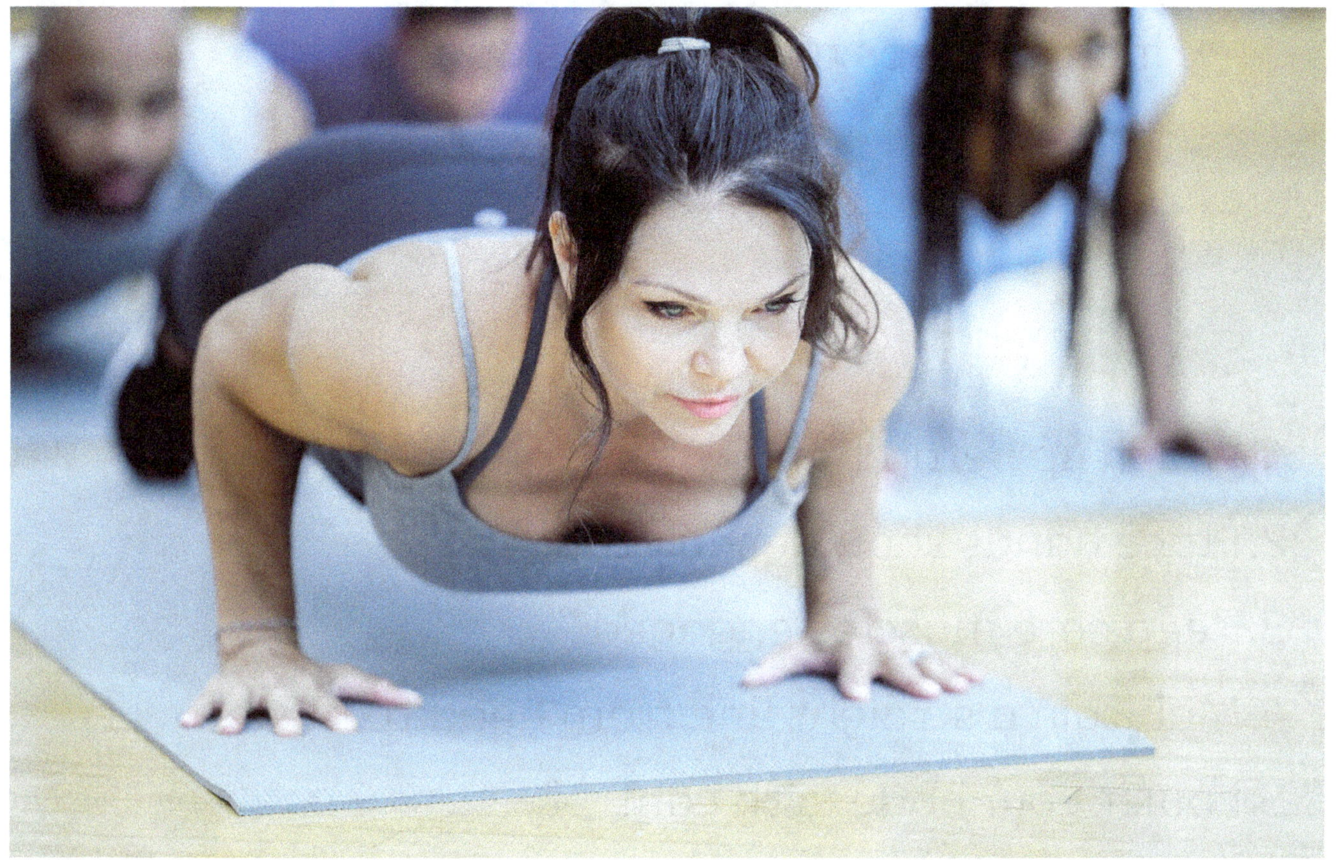

INSTRUCTIONS

- Get into a plank position.

- Hands shoulder-width apart.

- Lower body until elbows at 90 degrees.

- Keep back straight, core engaged.

- Push back up to starting position.

- Breathe out on the way up.

- Start with a comfortable number.
- Increase reps as strength improves.

SAFETY TIPS

1. Warm up beforehand.

2. Place hands shoulder-width apart.

3. Keep core muscles engaged.

4. Maintain a straight line from head to heels.

5. Lower your body with control.

6. Avoid sagging or arching your back.

7. Exhale as you push back up.

8. Listen to your body and avoid overdoing it.

REVERSE CRUNCHES

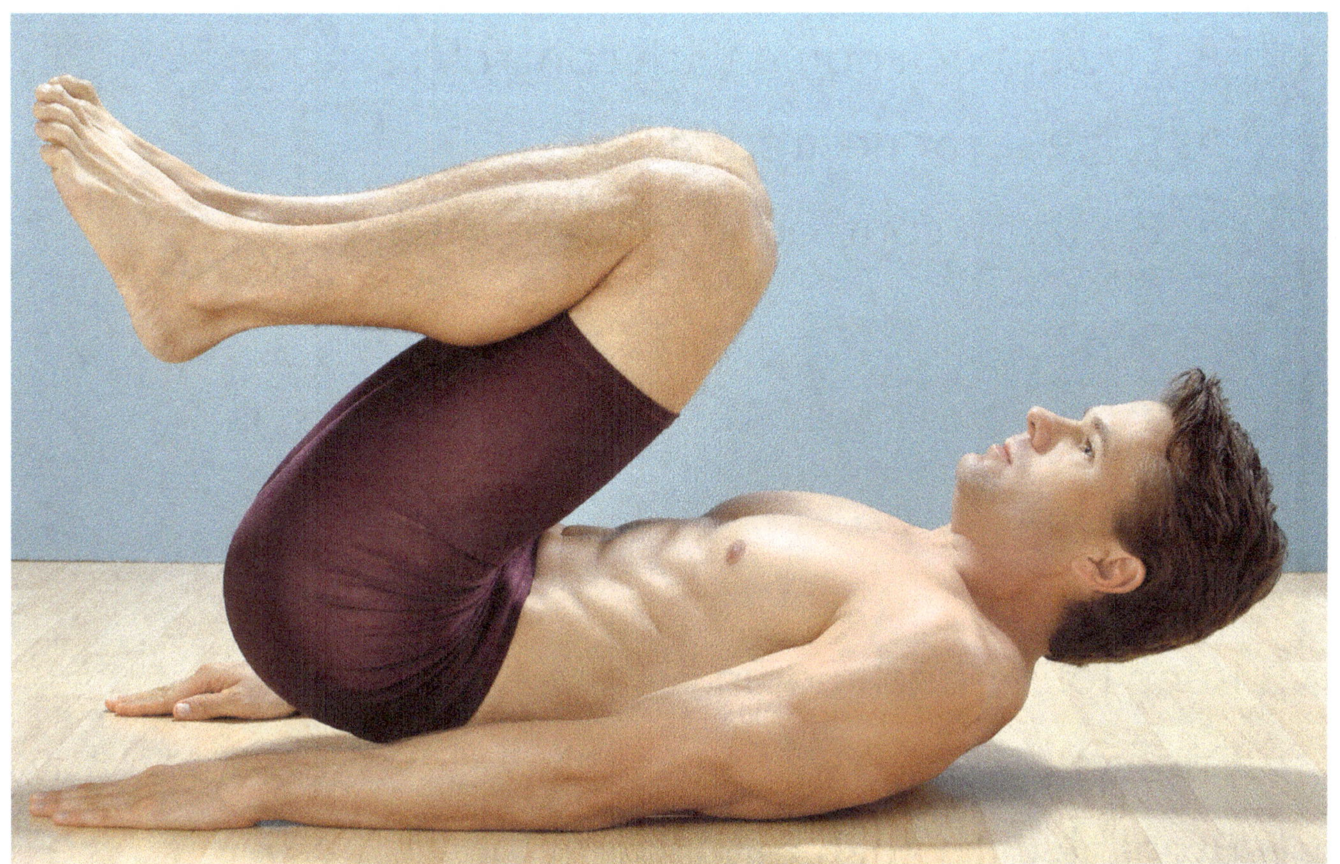

INSTRUCTIONS

- Lie flat on your back.

- Bend your knees at a 90-degree angle.

- Place hands flat on the floor or under your hips for support.

- Contract your abs to lift your hips off the floor.

- Bring your knees towards your chest.

- Lower back down with control.

- Repeat for desired reps.

- Focus on controlled movements.

SAFETY TIPS

1. Warm up.

2. Use a mat.

3. Keep lower back down.

4. Engage core.

5. Breathe with each movement.

6. Start with small movements.

7. Listen to your body.

LONG ARM CRUNCHES

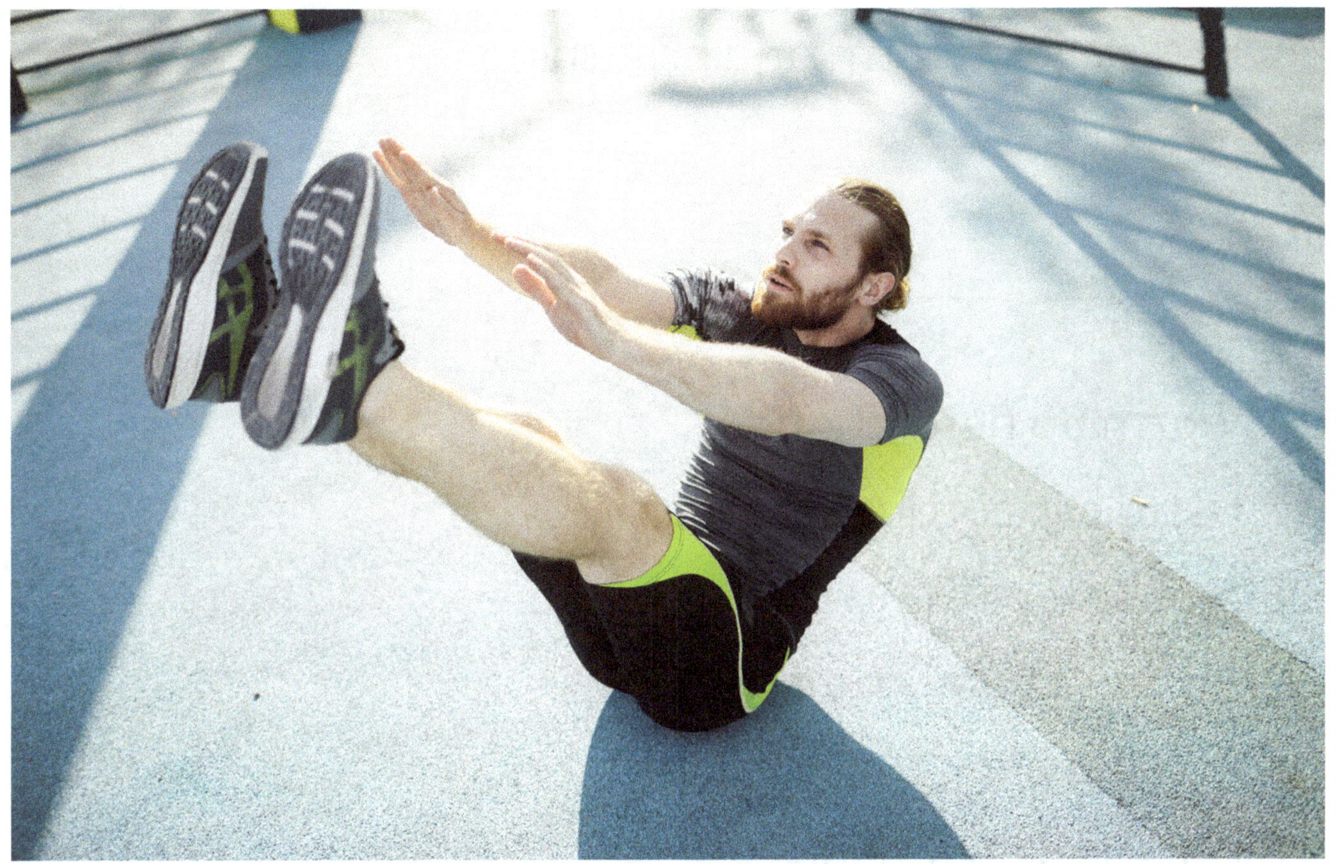

INSTRUCTIONS

- Lie flat on your back.

- Extend arms straight above head.

- Lift shoulders off the ground.

- Keep arms long and reach towards toes.

- Engage core muscles.

- Lower back down with control.

- Repeat for desired reps.
- Focus on form and breathing.

SAFETY TIPS

1. Warm up beforehand.
2. Use a supportive surface.
3. Move slowly and with control.
4. Exhale as you crunch up.
5. Avoid pulling on your neck.
6. Listen to your body.

BICYCLE CRUNCHES

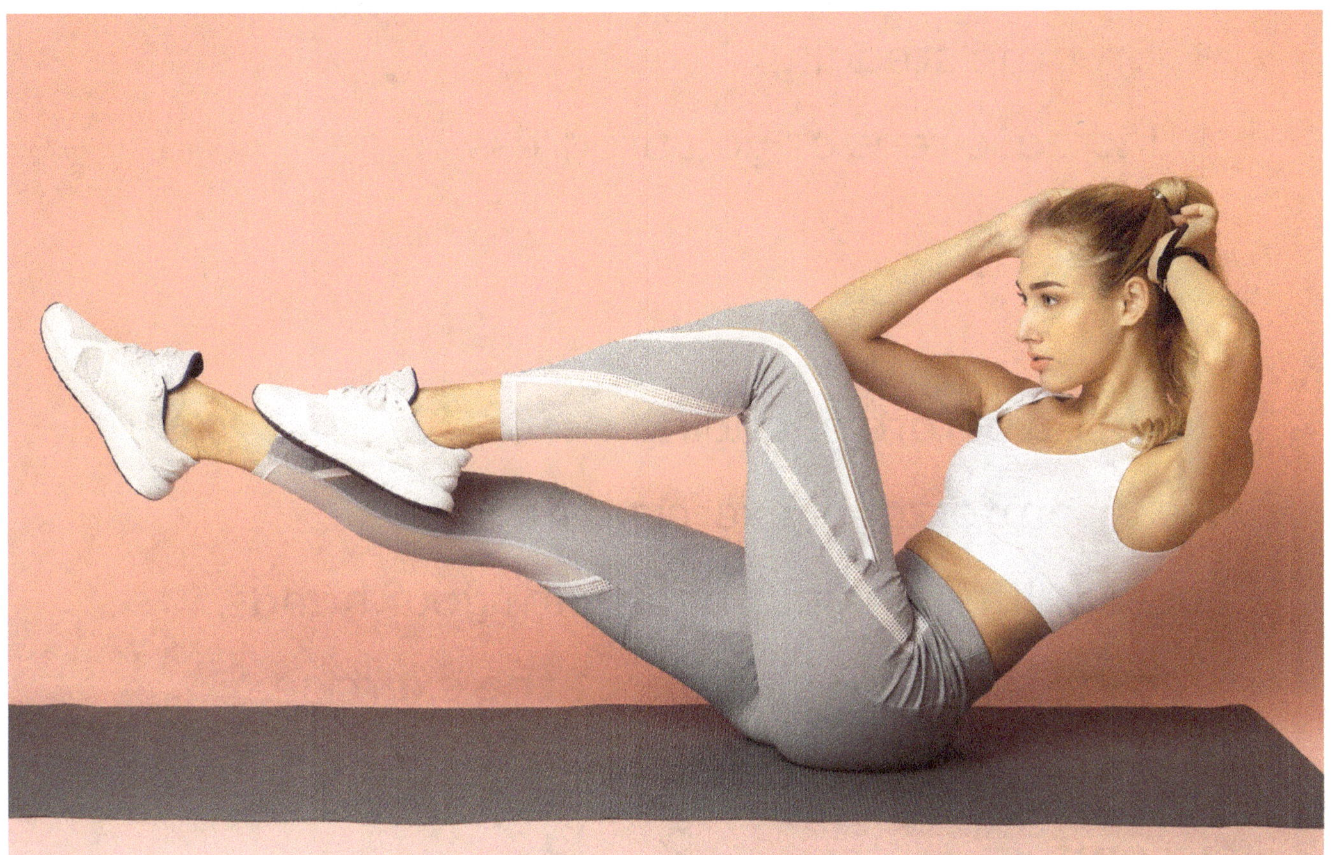

INSTRUCTIONS

- Lie on your back.

- Lift legs and bend knees.

- Place hands behind head.

- Alternate touching elbows to opposite knees.

- Extend legs out for extra challenge.

- Keep core engaged throughout.

- Aim for controlled movements.
- Breathe steadily.
- Increase reps as you progress.

SAFETY TIPS

1. Warm up before engaging
2. Use a comfortable exercise mat.
3. Avoid pulling on your neck with your hands.
4. Breathe steadily throughout the exercise.
5. Listen to your body and stop if you feel any discomfort.

JUMP SQUAT

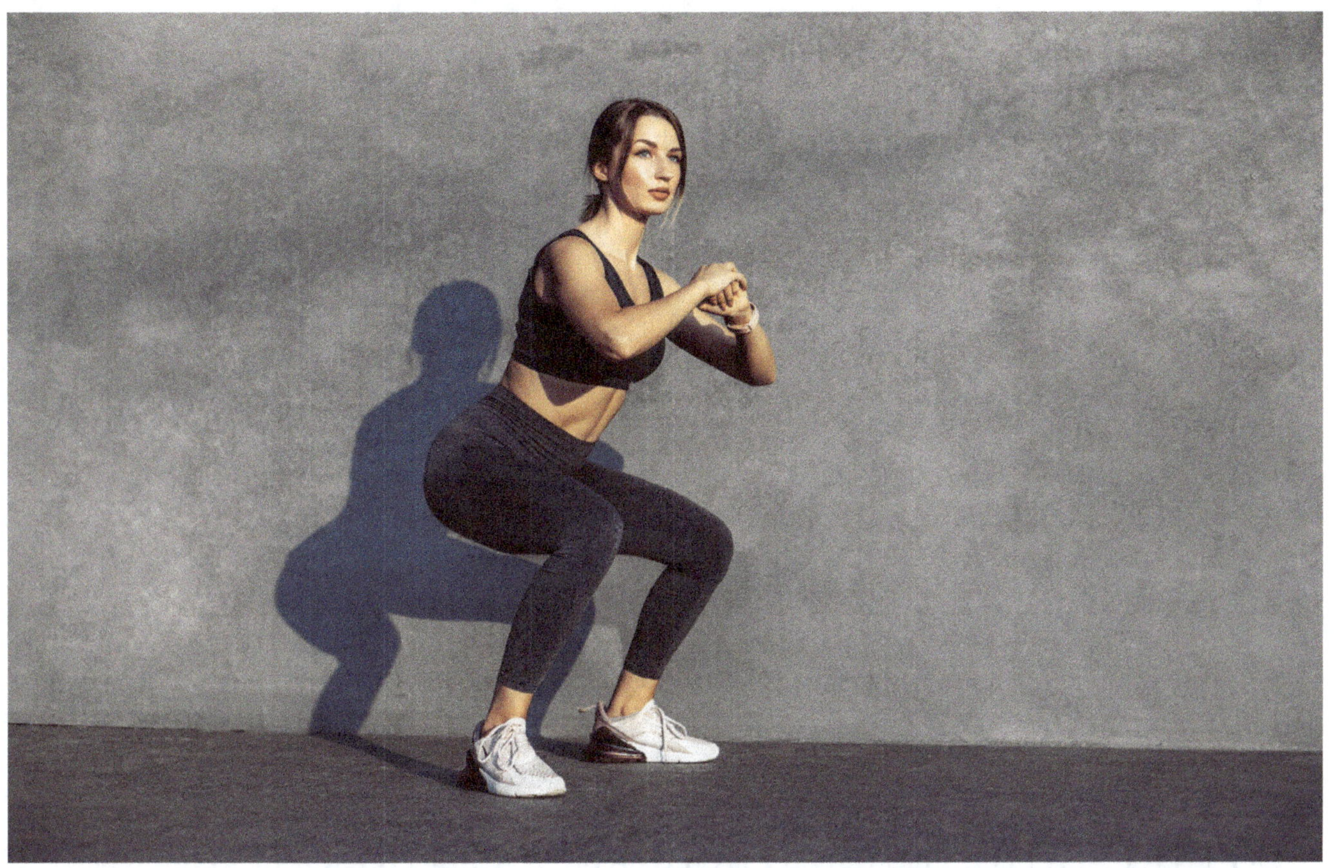

INSTRUCTIONS

- Stand as you would for a bodyweight squat, then push your back back and lower to a three-quarter squat depth position.

- As you lower down, move your arms down to your sides to 'load up' for your leap.

- Jump straight up, achieving triple-extension at the ankle, knee, and hips, swinging your arms up to help create momentum.

SAFETY TIPS

1. Warm up before starting jump squats.
2. Wear supportive athletic shoes.
3. Use a flat, non-slip surface for your workout.
4. Engage your core muscles throughout the exercise.
5. Explosively jump upwards, extending your legs fully.
6. Land softly, bending your knees to absorb the impact.
7. Keep your back straight and chest lifted throughout the movement.
8. Maintain a consistent rhythm and pace.
9. Listen to your body and take breaks if needed.

AIR SQUATS

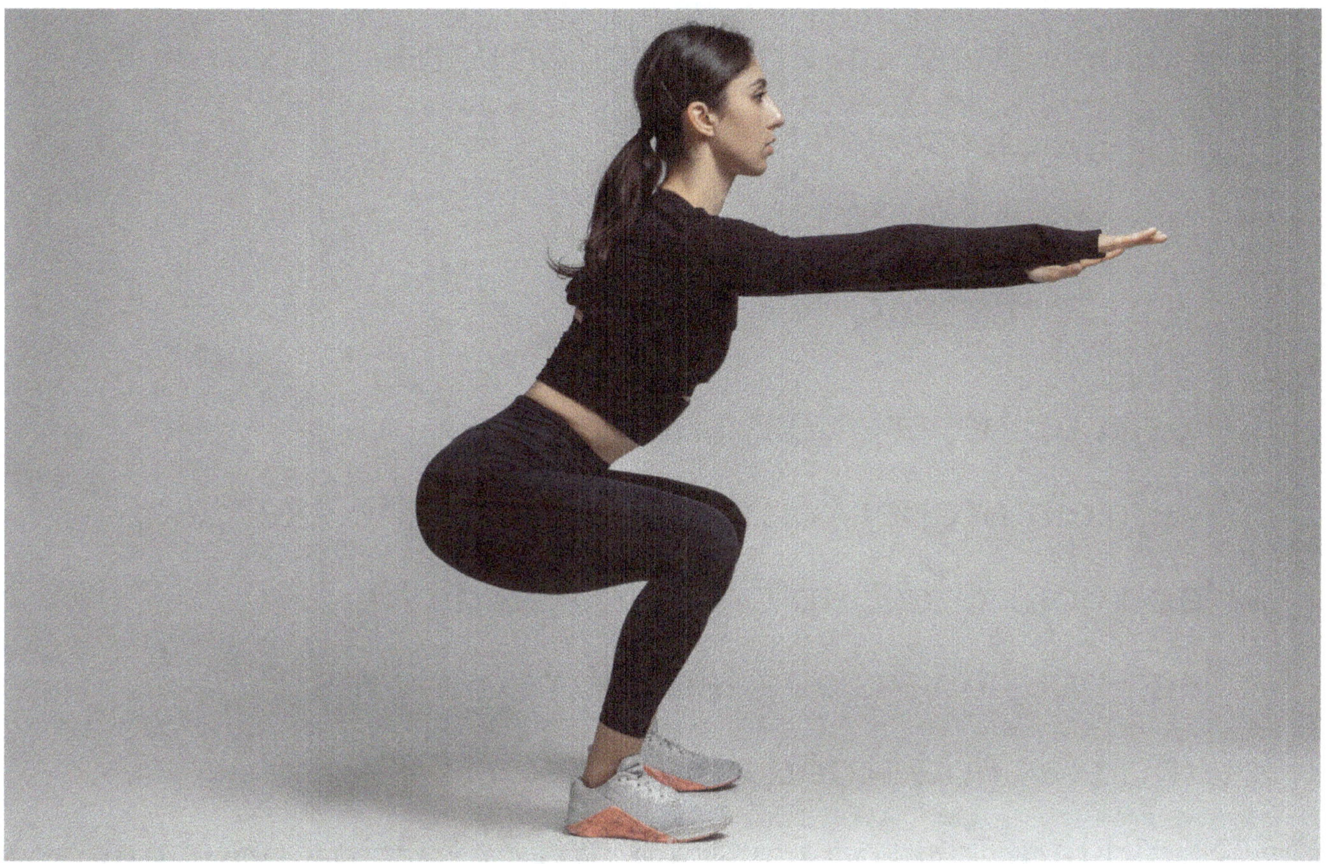

INSTRUCTIONS

- Stand with feet shoulder-width apart.
- Lower into a squat, keeping back straight.
- Hips go back and down.
- Knees track over toes.
- Lower until thighs are parallel to ground.
- Push through heels to stand.

- Engage core throughout.
- Keep chest up and gaze forward.
- Repeat for desired reps.

SAFETY TIPS

1. Warm up before doing air squats.
2. Maintain proper form throughout the exercise.
3. Keep your chest up and back straight.
4. Keep your knees aligned with your toes.
5. Exhale as you stand up.
6. Avoid leaning too far forward or letting your knees collapse inward.
7. Listen to your body

FROGGY JUMPS

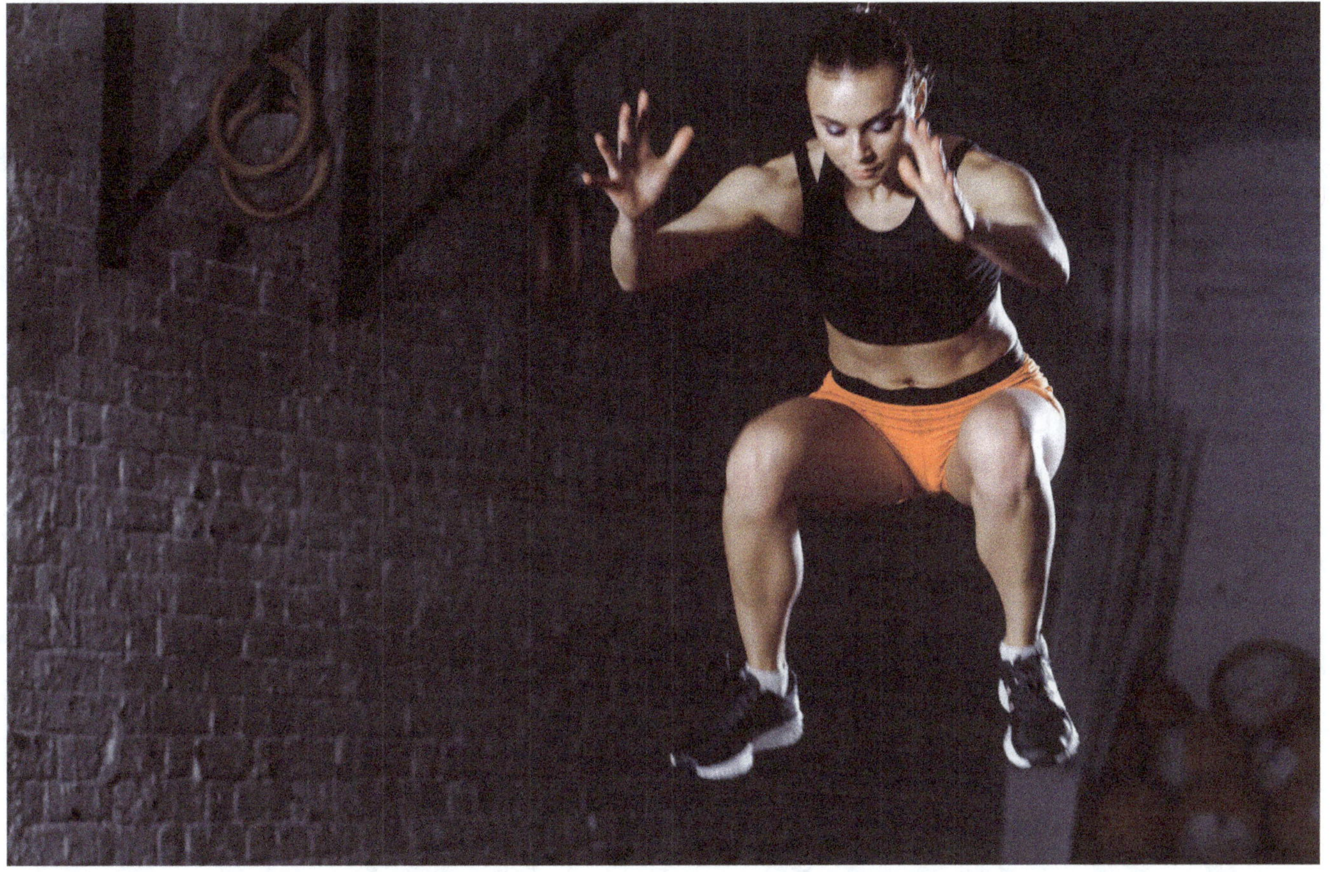

INSTRUCTIONS

- Start in a squat position.

- Explode upwards into a jump.

- Extend arms overhead.

- Land softly back into squat.

- Repeat in quick succession.

- Engage core muscles throughout.

- Aim for full range of motion.
- Increase speed for intensity.

SAFETY TIPS

1. Warm up beforehand.
2. Use a cushioned surface.
3. Land softly, bending your knees.
4. Keep your back straight.
5. Avoid locking your knees upon landing.
6. Listen to your body.

SLED PUSHES/PULLS

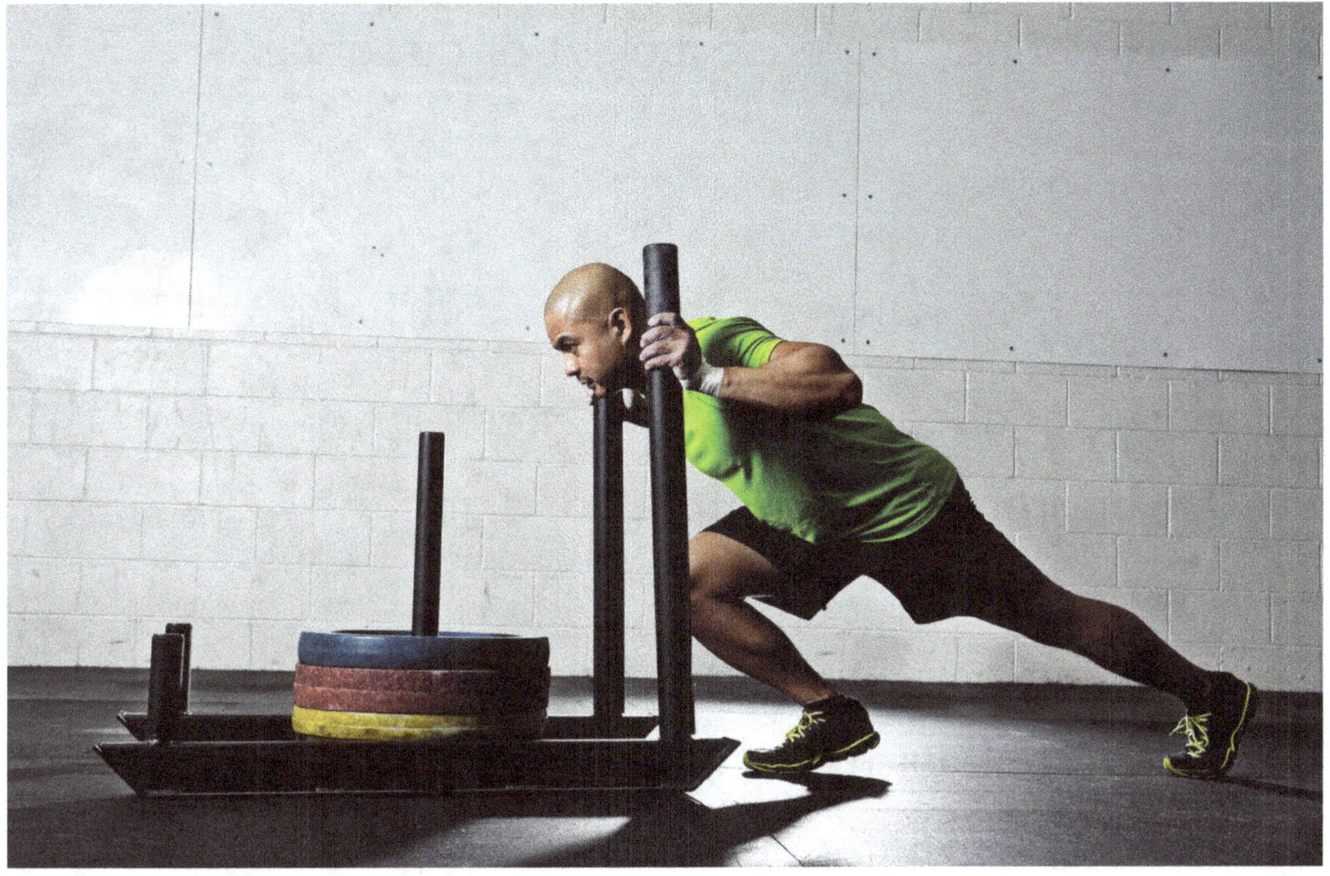

INSTRUCTIONS

- Set up sled with desired weight.

- Push sled forward with legs.

- Keep back straight, engage core.

- Use arms to stabilize and steer.

- Push explosively for short distances.

- Pull sled backward for variation.

- Focus on proper form and breathing.
- Gradually increase weight or distance.

SAFETY TIPS

1. Warm up adequately before sled work.
2. Use proper footwear with good grip.
3. Ensure the sled's path is clear.
4. Maintain a strong, stable posture.
5. Push or pull with controlled movements.
6. Watch your footing to prevent slipping.
7. Listen to your body

BEAR CRAWLS

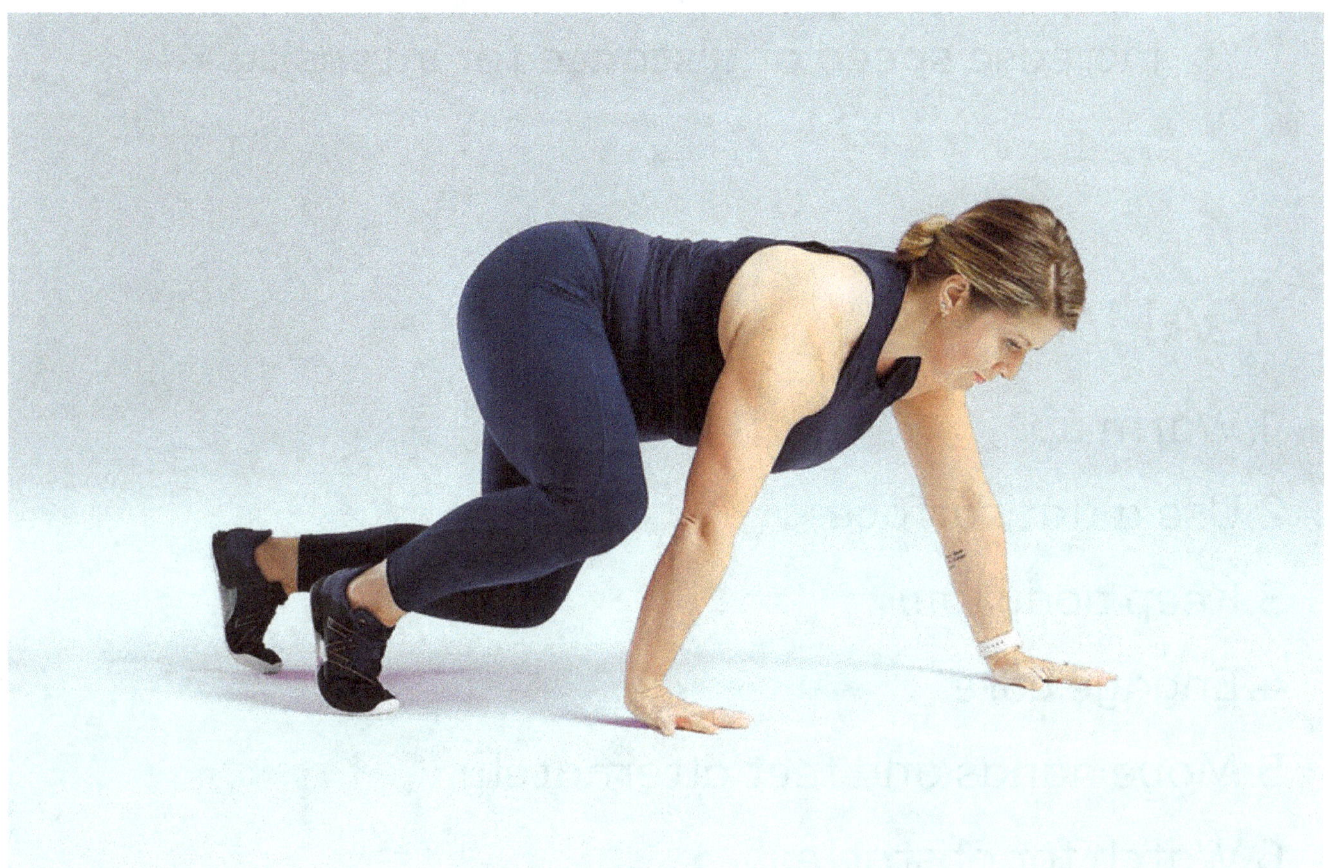

INSTRUCTIONS

- Get into a tabletop position on the floor.

- Lift knees slightly off the ground.

- Crawl forward with opposite hand and foot.

- Keep back flat and core engaged.

- Move slowly and steadily.

- Aim for controlled movements.

- Keep neck aligned with spine.
- Increase speed or distance for intensity.

SAFETY TIPS

1. Warm up.
2. Use a flat surface.
3. Keep body low.
4. Engage core.
5. Move hands and feet alternately.
6. Watch for obstacles.
7. Start slow.
8. Listen to your body.

PLANK JACKS

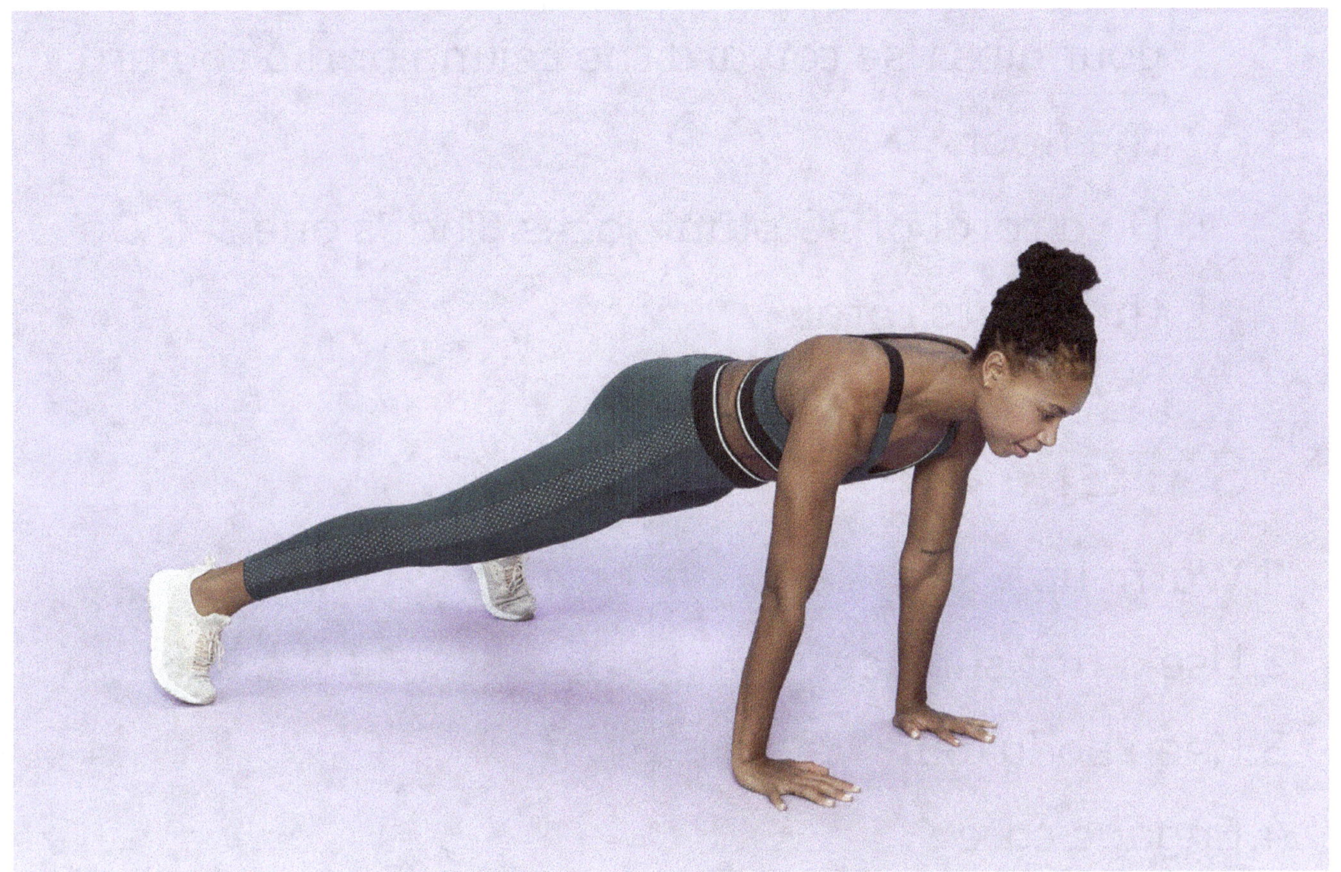

INSTRUCTIONS

- Start in plank position with your shoulders over your wrists, your body in one straight line, and your feet together.

- Like the motion of a jumping jack, jump your feet out wide and then back together.

- Try to keep your pelvis steady and don't let your hips rise toward the ceiling or dip toward the floor.
- Do a total of 30 plank jacks. That's one set. Do three sets total.

SAFETY TIPS

1. Warm up.
2. Use a flat surface.
3. Keep body low.
4. Engage core.
5. Move hands and feet alternately.
6. Watch for obstacles.
7. Start slow.
8. Listen to your body.

TRAMPOLINE JUMPING

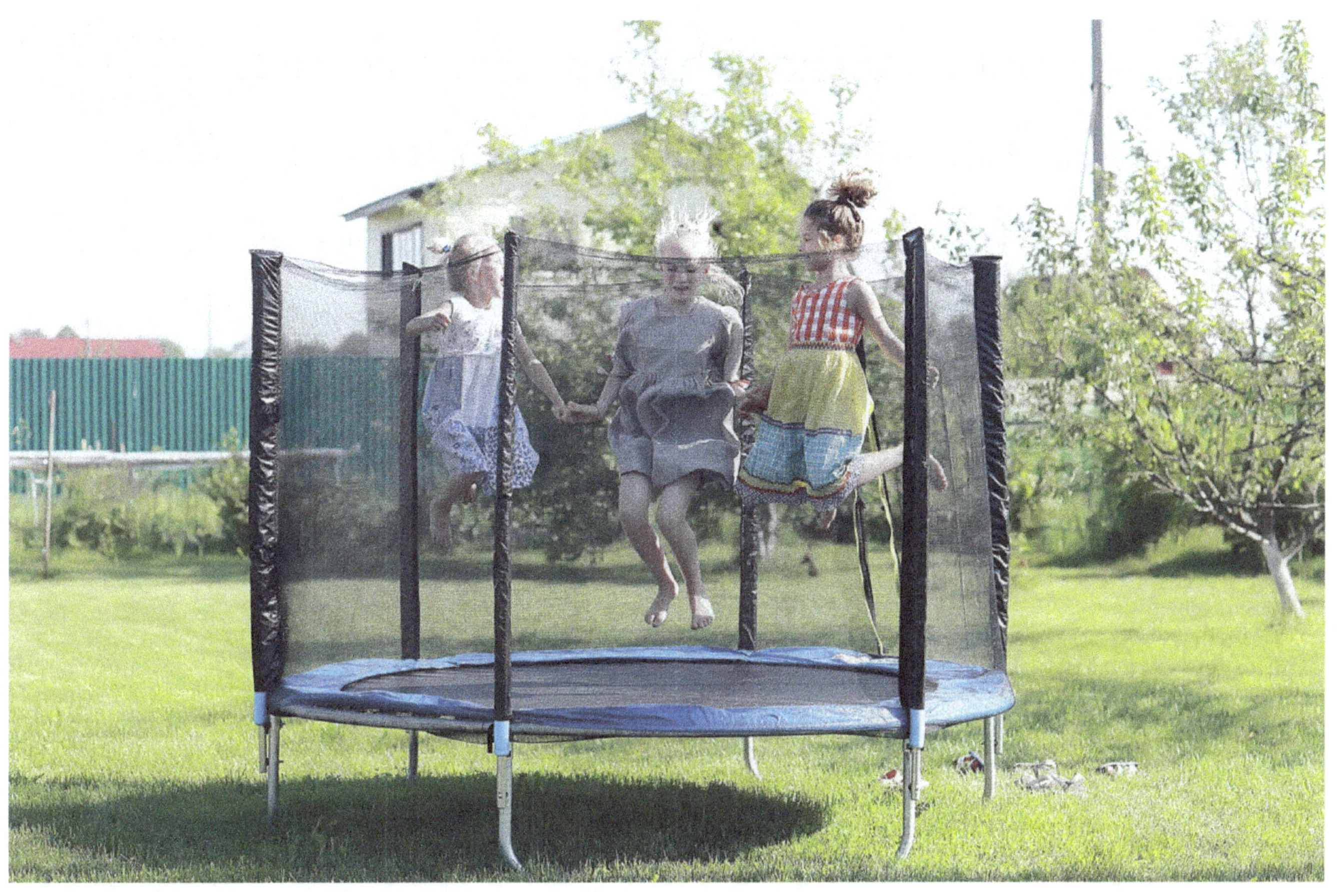

INSTRUCTIONS

- Find a suitable trampoline with safety netting.
- Step onto the trampoline with bare feet or non-slip socks.
- Bend your knees slightly to absorb the bounce.
- Use your arms for balance and momentum.

- Start with small jumps to get comfortable.

- Gradually increase height and intensity.

- Keep your jumps controlled and land softly.

- Try different movements like twists or tucks.

SAFETY TIPS

1. Warm up.

2. Avoid jumping too close to the edge.

3. Use a trampoline with safety netting.

4. Wear non-slip socks.

5. Jump in the center of the trampoline.

6. Avoid somersaults without proper training.

7. Stay aware of surroundings.

8. Exit carefully to avoid falls.

9. Take breaks to prevent fatigue.

10. Listen to your body for any discomfort.

TUCK JUMPS

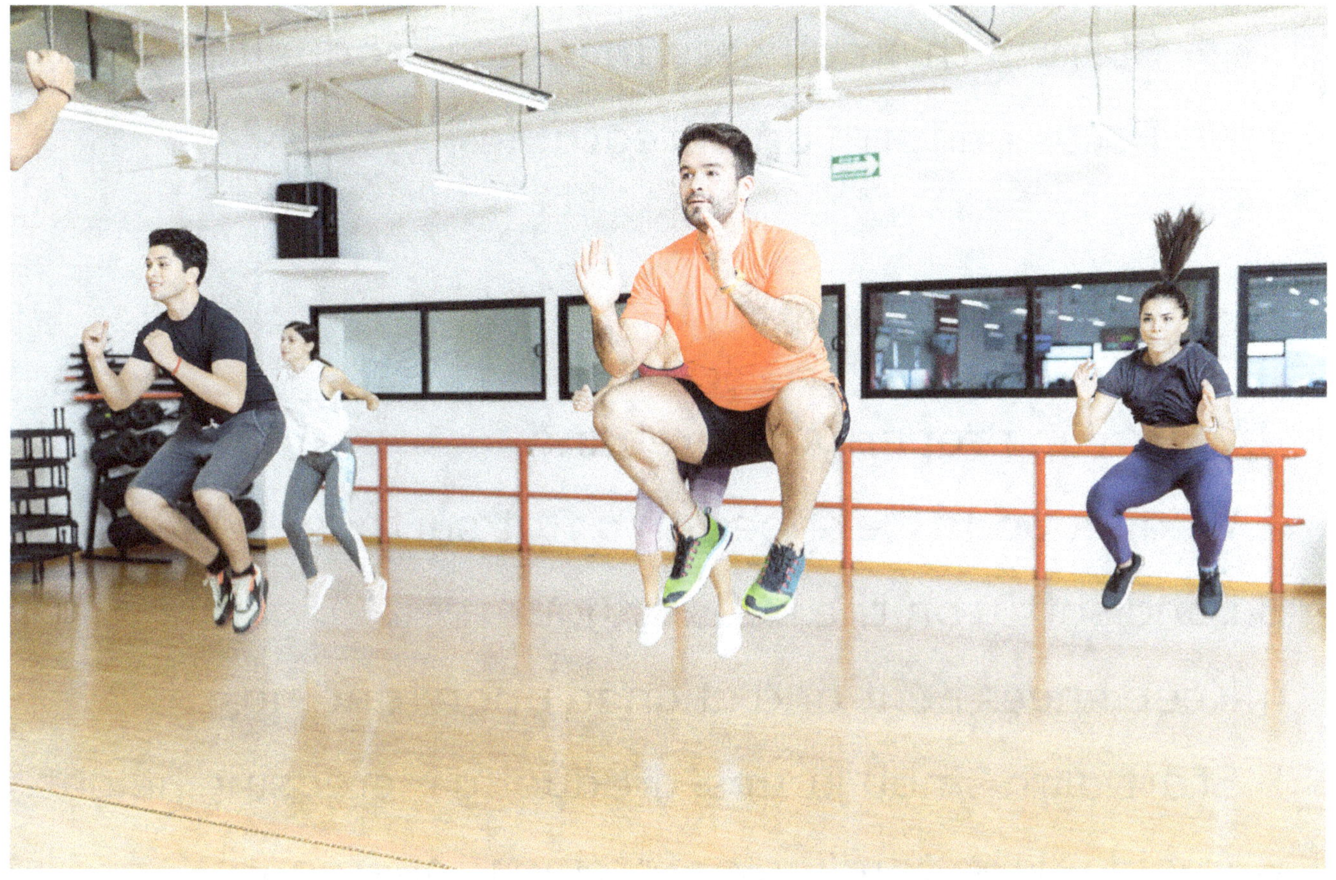

INSTRUCTIONS

- Stand with feet hip-width apart.
- Bend knees and jump upward.
- Bring knees toward chest.
- Extend legs before landing.
- Land softly with bent knees.
- Repeat in a controlled rhythm.

- Engage core for balance.
- Start with small sets, increase gradually.
- Focus on form and breathing.

SAFETY TIPS

1. Warm up properly beforehand.
2. Wear supportive shoes on a flat surface.
3. Land softly on the balls of your feet.
4. Keep knees bent and aligned upon landing.
5. Start with small jumps, gradually increasing height.
6. Avoid overextending or forcing movements.
7. Listen to your body and avoid overdoing it.

ADVANCED LEVEL

SPRINT INTERVALS

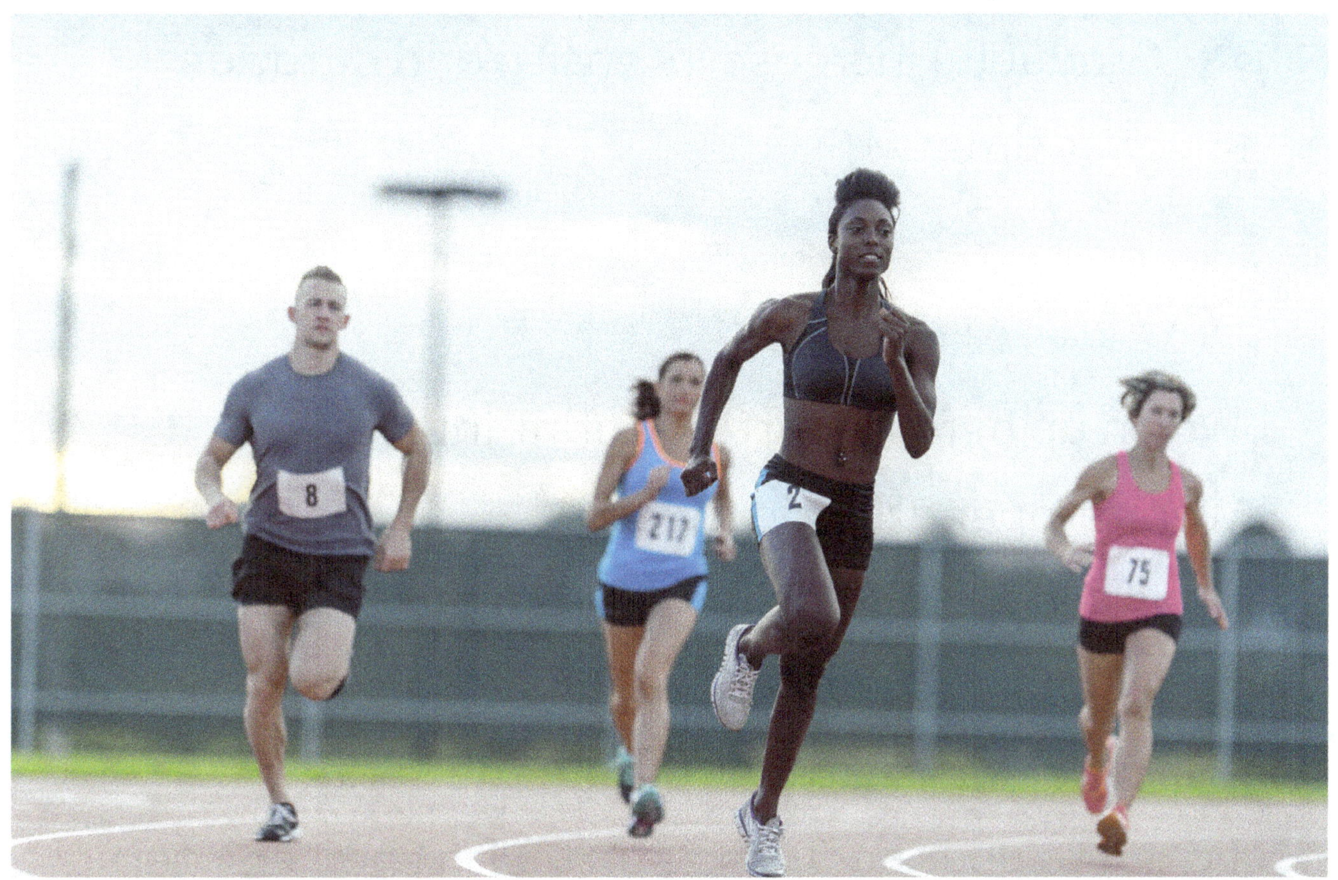

INSTRUCTIONS

- Find a flat, open space.

- Warm up with light jogging.

- Sprint at maximum effort for 20-30 seconds.

- Walk or jog for 60-90 seconds to recover.

- Repeat for 5-10 intervals.

- Cool down with a light jog or walk.

- Stay hydrated and listen to your body.
- Gradually increase intensity and duration over time.

SAFETY TIPS

1. Warm up before starting sprint intervals.
2. Wear proper athletic shoes.
3. Choose a flat, clear surface for sprinting.
4. Keep your body upright and maintain good posture.
5. Use short, quick strides during the sprint.
6. Listen to your body and start with shorter intervals.
7. Stay hydrated by drinking water before and after.
8. Pay attention to your surroundings to avoid obstacles.

PLYOMETRIC BOX JUMPS

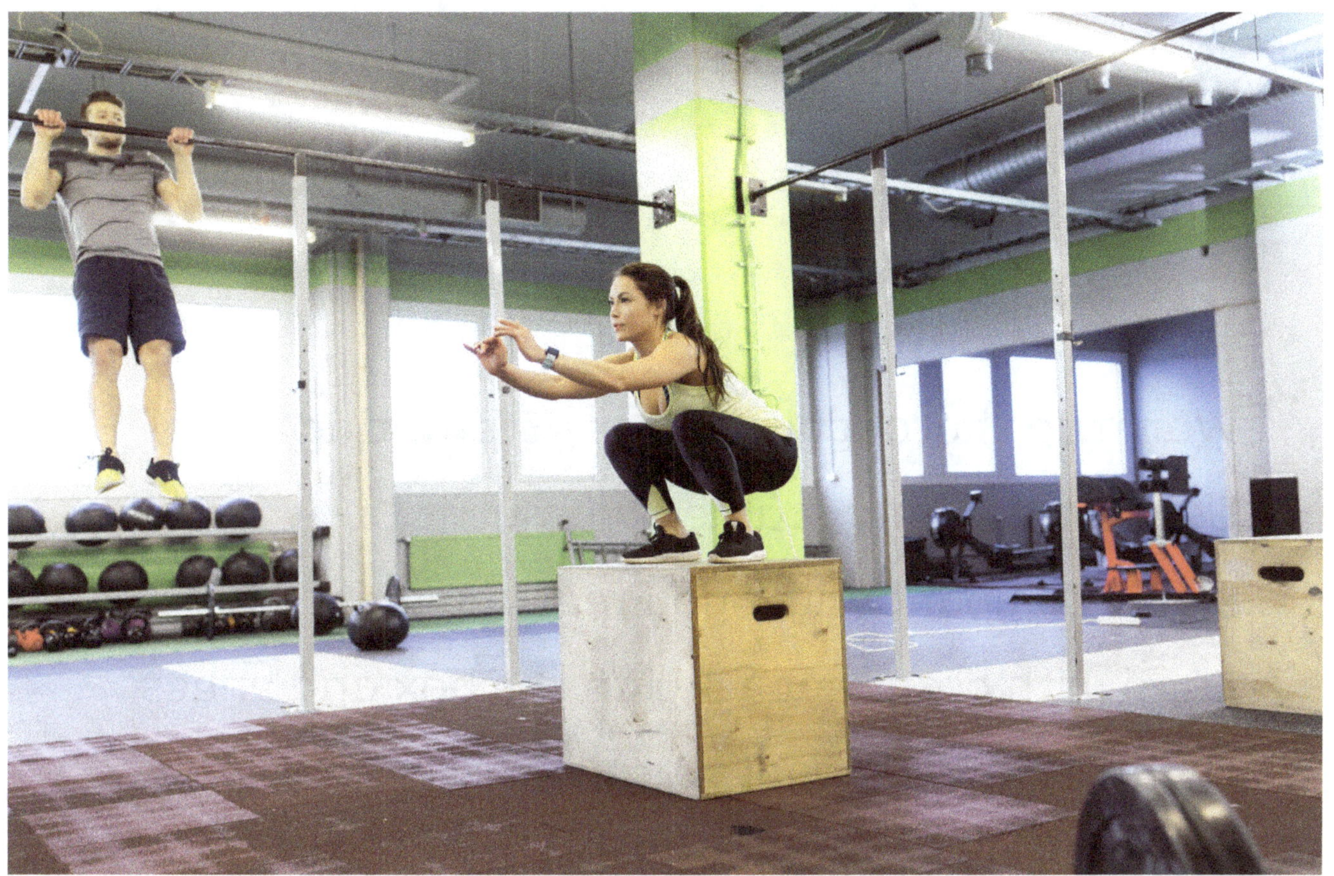

INSTRUCTIONS

- Find a plyo box of appropriate height.
- Stand in front with feet shoulder-width apart.
- Bend knees slightly, swing arms back.
- Explode upwards, swinging arms forward.
- Land softly on the box, knees bent.
- Step or jump back down.

- Start with a lower box height.
- Increase height gradually as strength improves.

SAFETY TIPS

1. Warm up thoroughly before attempting
2. Use a sturdy and stable plyometric box.
3. Listen to your body if you feel any pain
4. Land with both feet fully on the box and knees slightly bent to absorb impact.
5. Avoid locking your knees upon landing to prevent injury.

BATTLE ROPES

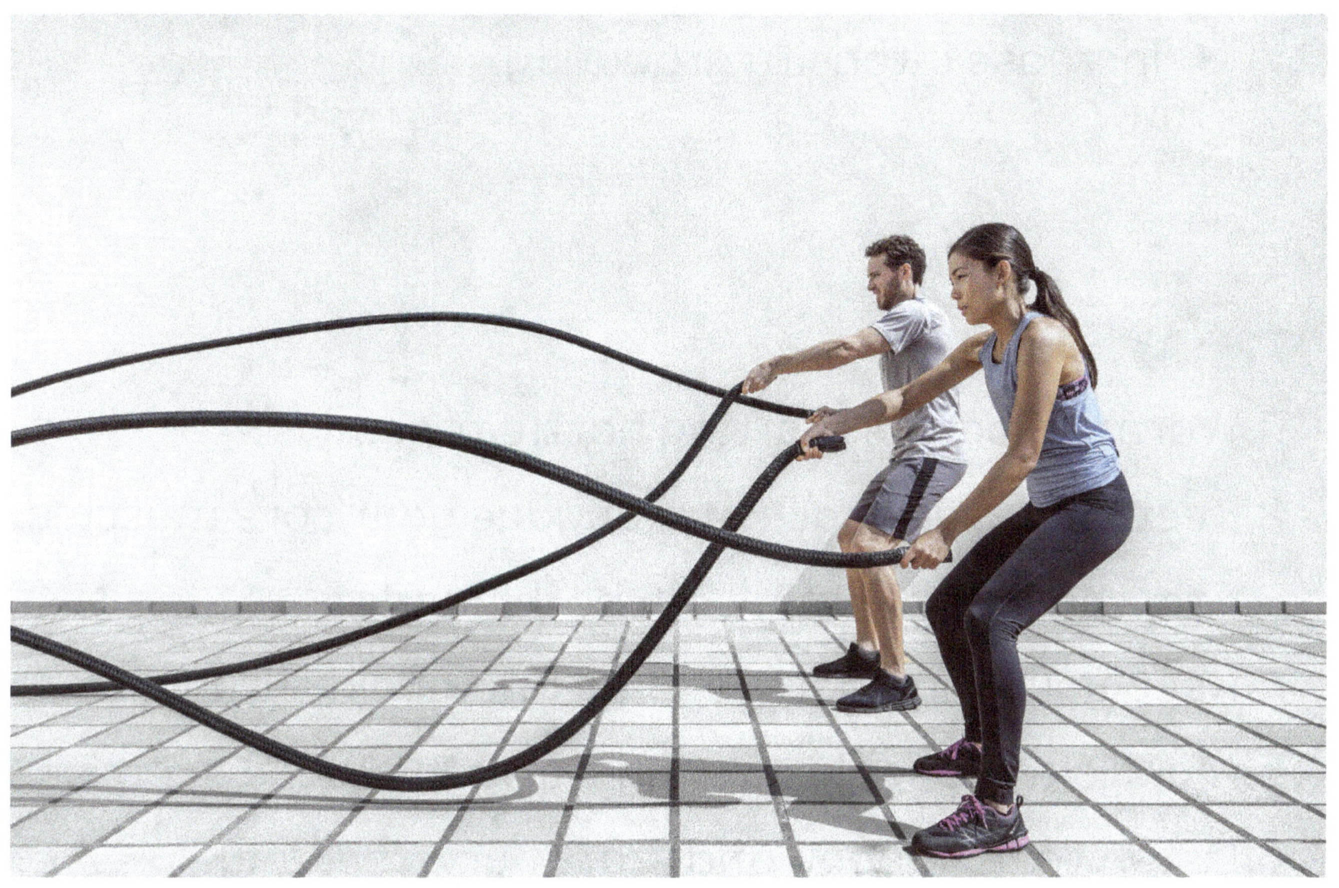

INSTRUCTIONS

- Secure battle ropes to anchor point.

- Stand with feet shoulder-width apart.

- Hold one end of each rope in each hand.

- Move arms simultaneously up and down.

- Generate waves or slams.

- Keep core engaged for stability.

- Start with shorter intervals.
- Increase intensity gradually.

SAFETY TIPS

1. Warm up before starting battle ropes.
2. Keep a straight back and engage your core muscles.
3. Grip the ropes firmly with both hands.
4. Keep your shoulders relaxed and avoid shrugging.
5. Maintain proper breathing throughout the exercise.
6. Listen to your body and stop if you feel any discomfort.

KETTLEBELL SWINGS

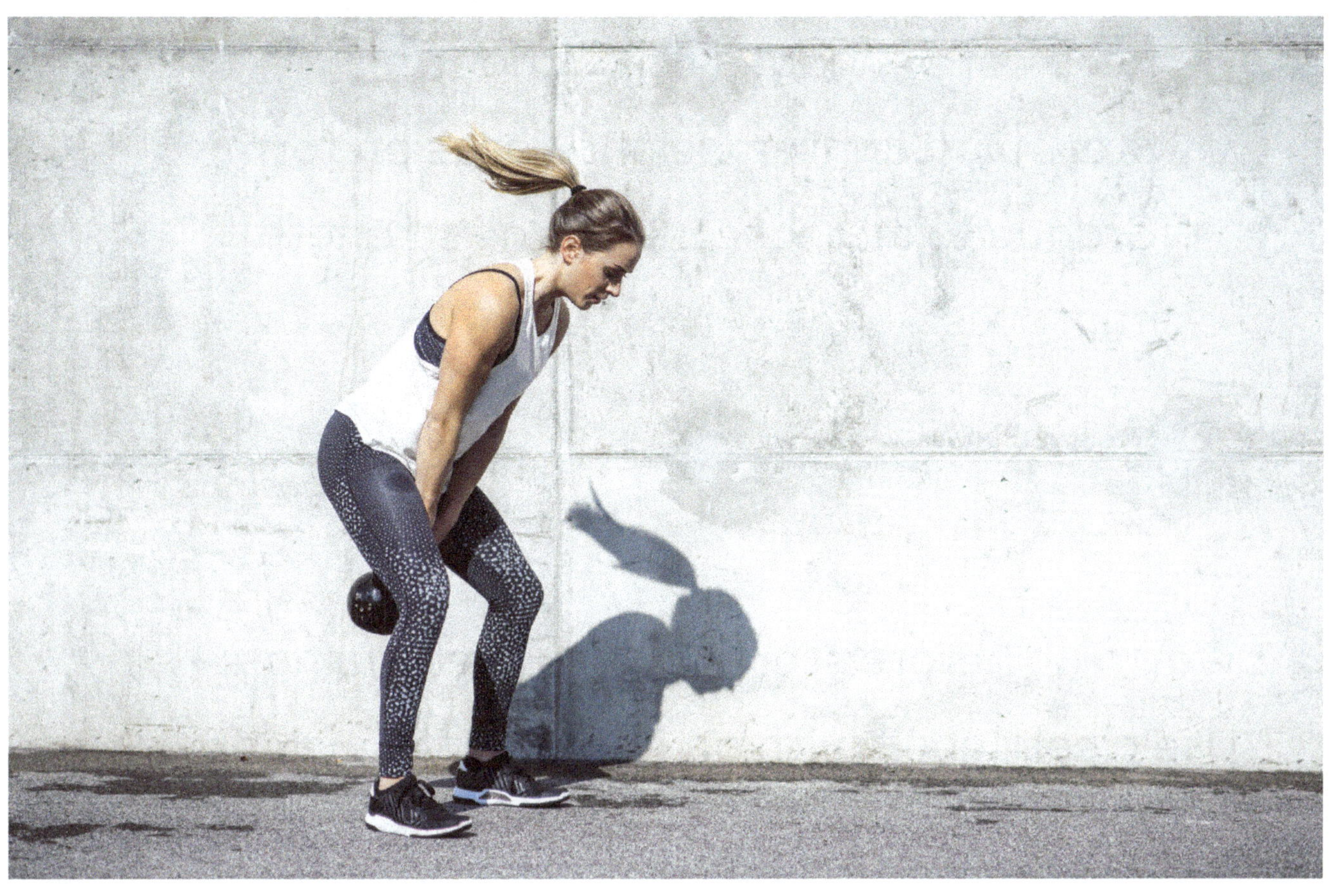

INSTRUCTIONS

- Stand with feet shoulder-width apart.

- Hold kettlebell with both hands between legs.

- Hinge at hips, keeping back straight.

- Swing kettlebell forcefully up to shoulder height.

- Use hips, not arms, for power.

- Control the swing on the way down.
- Keep core engaged throughout.
- Start with lighter weight, focus on form.
- Gradually increase weight as strength improves.

SAFETY TIPS

1. Warm up before starting kettlebell swings.
2. Use a kettlebell with an appropriate weight
3. Stand with feet shoulder-width apart and grip the kettlebell handle.
4. Keep your arms straight and relaxed, letting the kettlebell swing naturally.
5. Avoid arching your back or rounding your shoulders at the top of the swing.
6. Keep breathing throughout the movement, exhaling on the upswing and inhaling on the downswing.
7. Stop immediately if you feel any pain or discomfort.

ROWING SPRINTS

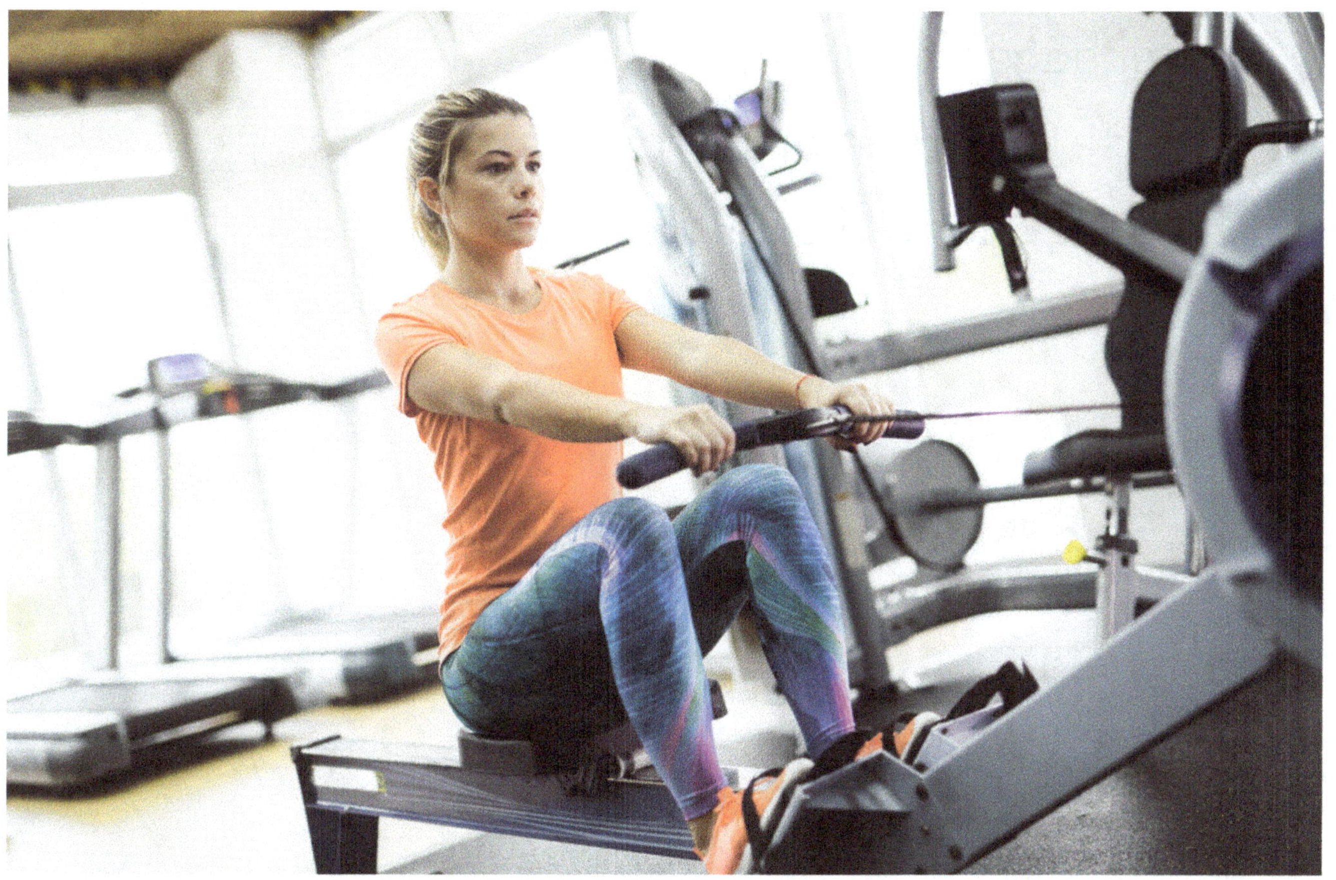

INSTRUCTIONS

- Set up rowing machine.

- Sit with feet strapped in.

- Grab handle with overhand grip.

- Push off with legs, then pull handle towards chest.

- Row explosively for short bursts.

- Maintain proper form: back straight, core engaged.
- Use legs, then arms for power.
- Rest briefly between sprints.

SAFETY TIPS

1. Warm up.
2. Secure feet in straps.
3. Sit tall with straight back.
4. Engage core.
5. Control breathing.
6. Avoid hyperextending knees.
7. Maintain proper form.
8. Listen to your body.

AGILITY LADDER DRILLS

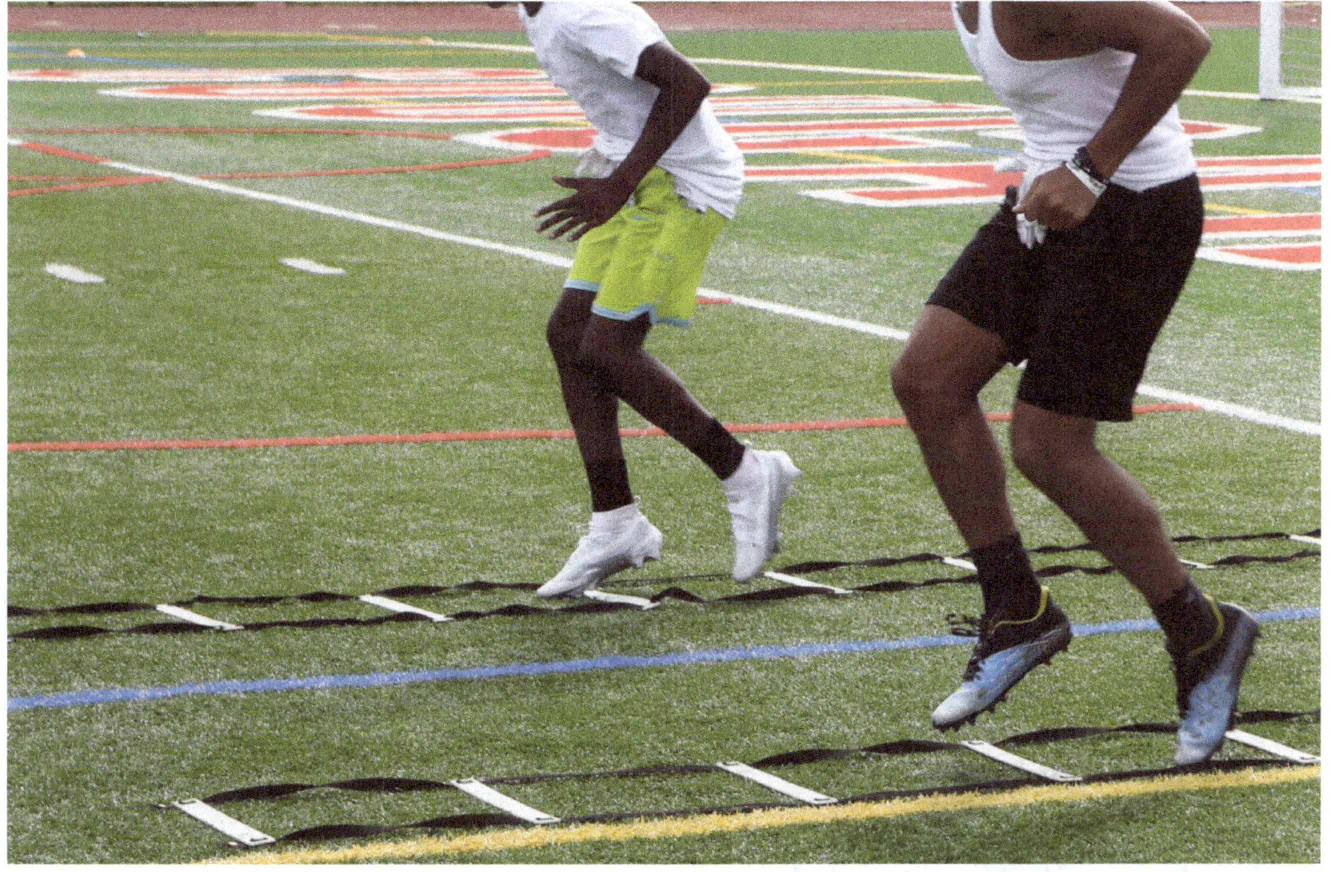

INSTRUCTIONS

- Lay out an agility ladder flat on the ground.

- Stand at one end with feet hip-width apart.

- Step in and out of ladder squares quickly.

- Keep movements light and precise.

- Try various patterns like side steps, hops, and crosses.

- Focus on speed and coordination.
- Practice drills regularly to improve agility.
- Start with simple patterns and progress to more complex ones.

SAFETY TIPS

1. Warm up.
2. Wear good shoes.
3. Use a flat surface.
4. Start with basic drills.
5. Maintain proper form.
6. Keep movements light.
7. Engage core muscles.
8. Increase intensity gradually.
9. Take breaks as needed.
10. Cool down and stretch.

HILL SPRINTS

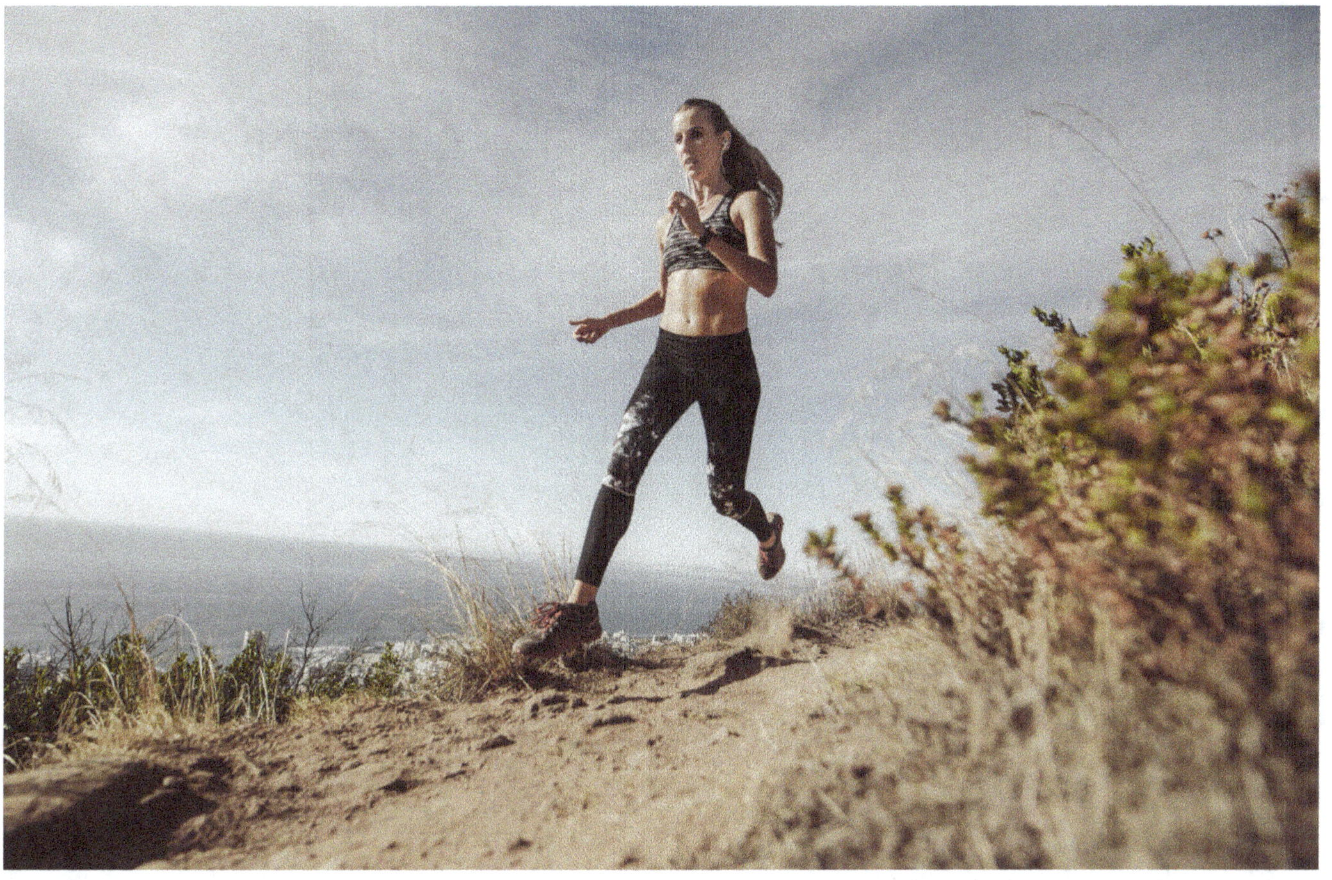

INSTRUCTIONS

- Find a steep hill.

- Warm up with light jogging.

- Sprint up the hill as fast as you can.

- Focus on driving knees and arms.

- Take shorter, quicker strides.

- Jog or walk back down for recovery.

- Start with a few sprints, gradually increase.
- Cool down with a light jog or walk.
- Stay hydrated and listen to your body.

SAFETY TIPS

1. Warm up properly.
2. Choose a safe hill.
3. Wear good shoes.
4. Maintain proper form.
5. Engage your core.
6. Use short, quick strides.
7. Listen to your body.
8. Cool down afterward.

SLAM BALL THROWS

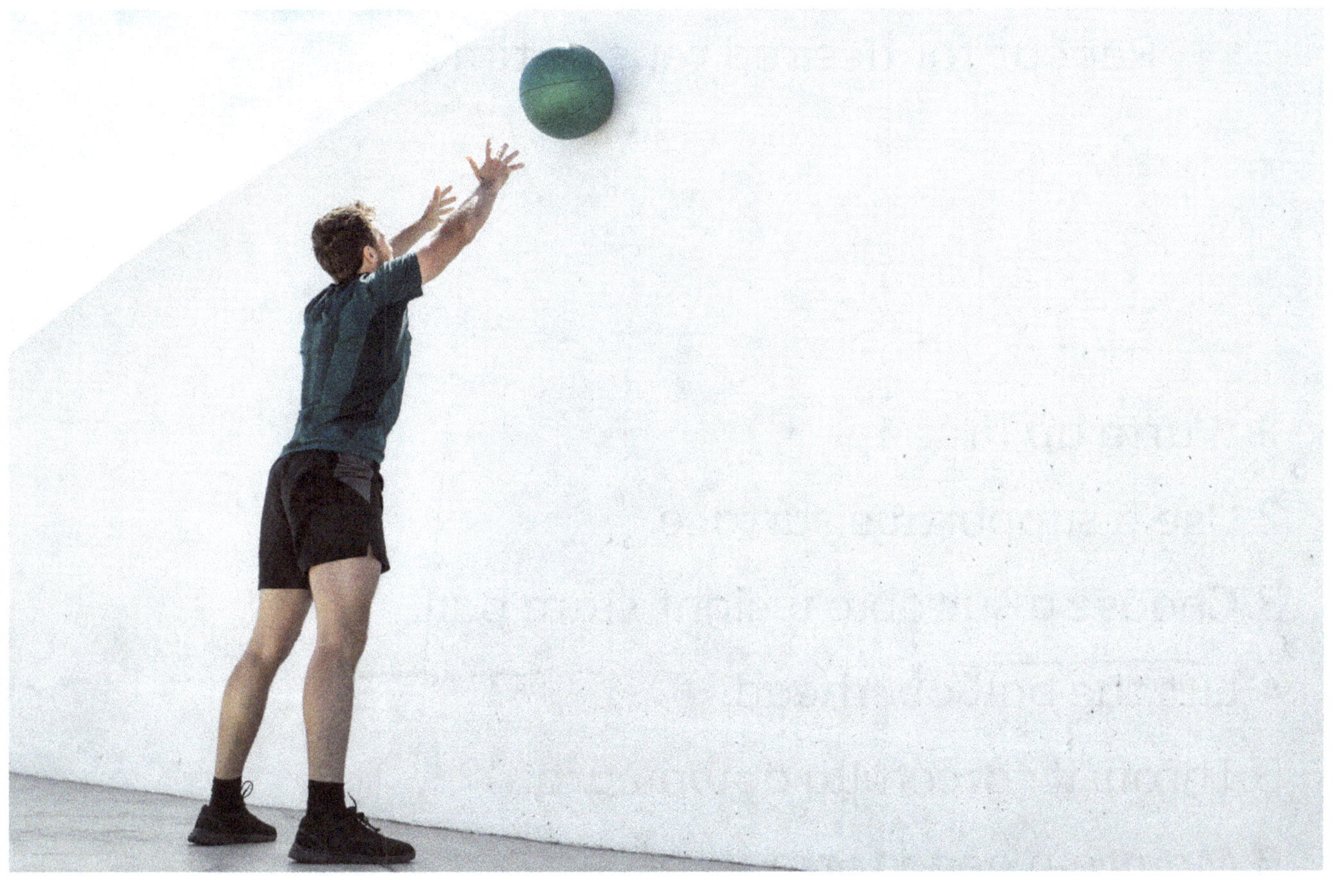

INSTRUCTIONS

- Choose a slam ball of appropriate weight.

- Stand with feet shoulder-width apart.

- Lift the slam ball above your head.

- Slam the ball down with force.

- Catch it on the bounce or pick it up.

- Engage your core throughout the motion.

- Use your whole body for power.
- Repeat for desired reps or time.

SAFETY TIPS

1. Warm up first.
2. Use a supportive surface.
3. Choose a suitable weight slam ball.
4. Lift the ball overhead.
5. Throw it forcefully downward.
6. Maintain good form.
7. Start with lighter weights.
8. Listen to your body.

TIRE FLIPS

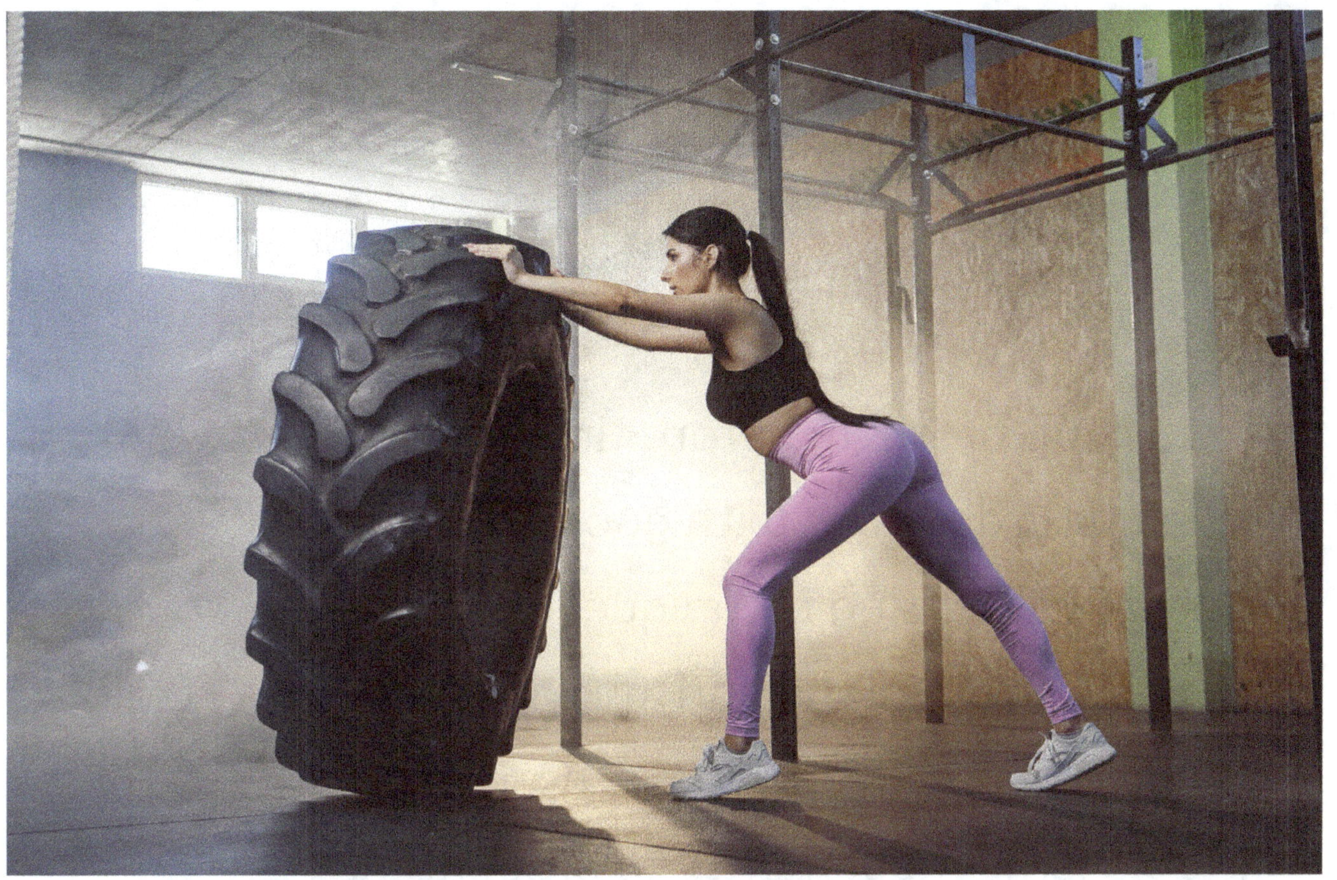

INSTRUCTIONS

- Find a sturdy tire.

- Stand behind it with feet shoulder-width apart.

- Squat down, grab the bottom of the tire.

- Lift with legs and flip the tire over.

- Use momentum to flip it quickly.

- Keep back straight, engage core.
- Repeat for desired reps or time.
- Rest as needed between sets.

SAFETY TIPS

1. Warm up properly before tire flips.
2. Wear sturdy shoes with good grip.
3. Use proper lifting technique.
4. Push with your legs and lift with your back straight.
5. Keep a firm grip on the tire handles.
6. Avoid jerky movements to prevent injury.
7. Listen to your body and take breaks as needed.

CONCLUSION

In summary, while somatic exercises may not directly target the heart muscle, they contribute to overall cardiovascular health by improving circulation, reducing stress, enhancing flexibility and range of motion, promoting body awareness, and supporting recovery and rehabilitation. Incorporating somatic exercises into a comprehensive approach to heart health can complement traditional cardiovascular exercise and lifestyle modifications, helping individuals achieve and maintain optimal cardiovascular well-being.